THE FIRST YEAR™

Hypothyroidism

An Essential Guide for the Newly Diagnosed

MAUREEN PRATT is a journalist and author whose work has appeared in the *Los Angeles Times, National Business Employment Weekly,* and other publications. She is coauthor of *Taking Charge of Lupus: How to Manage the Disease and Make the Most of Your Life* and is active nationally in raising awareness for thyroid disorders and lupus. Pratt lives in Los Angeles.

THE FIRST YEAR™

Hypothyroidism

An Essential Guide for the Newly Diagnosed

Maureen Pratt

Foreword by Elliot G. Levy, M.D.

MARLOWE & COMPANY ■ NEW YORK

THE FIRST YEAR™—HYPOTHYROIDISM:
An Essential Guide for the Newly Diagnosed
Copyright © 2003 by Maureen Pratt
Foreword copyright © 2003 by Elliot G. Levy, M.D.

Published by
Marlowe & Company
An Imprint of Avalon Publishing Group Incorporated
245 West 17th Street • 11th Floor
New York, NY 10011

The First Year™ and A Patient-Expert Walks You
Through Everything You Need to Learn and Do™ are
trademarks of the Avalon Publishing Group.

Library of Congress Cataloging-in-Publication Data is
available.

ISBN 1-56924-496-0

9   8   7   6   5   4

*Designed by Pauline Neuwirth,
   Neuwirth and Associates, Inc.*

Printed in the United States of America

Distributed by Publishers Group West

To Dorothy and Gertrude—
my two grandmothers—with whom
I shared much . . . even
thyroid disease!

Contents

CONTENTS

Foreword

by Elliot G. Levy, M.D.

DURING THE twenty-seven years that I have been in practice, many things have changed. In the "old days" of my parents' generation, a patient totally trusted his or her doctor. The family doctor was usually a well-revered general practitioner or internist and rarely, if ever, was anyone referred to a specialist. The doctor never gave a specific diagnosis; there was no questioning the doctor's decisions or choice of medications or other forms of treatment. There was no place to look up information about what was wrong—libraries were usually filled with outdated textbooks—and there were certainly no support groups to help people through an illness. The hospital was where we went if someone was sick, and it was hardly ever said that a bad outcome was a result of a bad doctor. Boy, are things different now.

The biggest change is the constant quest for knowledge and information that so many patients are on. I'm a specialist, so this means that I only see new patients who are referred for consultation and who already have or are suspected of having a thyroid problem. By the time I'm seeing a patient, they've already asked their doctor, their relatives, their friends, and their favorite search engine on the Internet for information about their condition. Often they come in with pages and pages of information they have downloaded from the Internet, sometimes from sites that I believe provide improper information. This makes my job more challenging than ever before. Not only do I have to be skilled at diagnosing a thyroid problem and figuring out the best treatment approach, now I have to explain through words, pictures, diagrams, and models exactly what is going on. We are truly in the Information Age, and I can use all the help I can get.

I have made it my mission to check out as many Web sites as possible and read as many books about thyroid disorders as I can find, both in bookstores and online. I need to know what my patients are reading so I can decide if the information provided is accurate and helpful or just a waste of their time. Some books are written for physicians, all very technical, scientific, and difficult to read, and are meant to be a resource for endocrinologists and scientists. Others are written by physicians for patients, giving thorough explanations for various thyroid diseases. And then there are the books written by patients trying to explain in lay terms their interpretation of thyroid problems. Unfortunately, many of these books revolve around the authors' unique experience with thyroid disease, and do not offer any real insight or advice to the average person with thyroid problems. Many of these books also carry an "anti-doctor" message, which is extremely unhealthy.

The First Year—Hypothyroidism by Maureen Pratt is unique. In these pages you will find medical information that has been thoroughly researched, discussed with experts from around the world, and is representative of the mainstream theories that exist in thyroidology. There are clear and detailed explanations of symptoms and how they relate to hypothyroidism. But most importantly, and completely unique to this book, *The First Year—Hypothyroidism* is set up to walk newly diagnosed readers through everything they need to know and do during the first seven days after diagnosis, then the next three weeks, and finally the next eleven months with hypothyroidism. In addition to giving you all the necessary medical information, Ms. Pratt helps you come to terms with living with symptoms that are hard to diagnose and talks about what it's like to experience changes in your symptoms as treatment starts to work for you. The sections about weight gain, hair loss, and depression are particularly important for thyroid patients to read and understand because Ms. Pratt is so realistic in her advice. Most books or articles claim that these conditions are clearly related to thyroid disease and will get better with treatment. But what happens if they don't? The emotional and psychological support provided in this book is outstanding. Ms. Pratt gives patients the motivation and often the courage to push on.

Some people are happy with just the explanation that their doctor provides about hypothyroidism. Some are satisfied with the information that a general thyroid Web site like the ones listed in the Resources section of this book can give. Other people want to know everything they can find out about hypothyroidism and read all the medical books and information out there on it. But most people want someone to hold their hand and guide them through the experience of being diagnosed and treated for hypothyroidism, and this is where Maureen Pratt comes in.

The First Year—Hypothyroidism is perfect for you if you're looking for a sympathetic ear and the support of someone who has suffered through everything that you are going through, someone who is willing to share with the world her life and her experiences with hypothyroidism.

ELLIOT G. LEVY, M.D., F.A.C.E. is a Clinical Professor of Medicine at the University of Miami School of Medicine. He lives in Miami, Florida.

Introduction

THIS BOOK is for anyone who has just been diagnosed with hypothyroidism. Whether you have Hashimoto's thyroiditis (an autoimmune disease) or another ailment that renders your thyroid gland underactive, this book will, I hope, give you some concrete information and suggestions about how to cope with this chronic illness and its related symptoms (including weight gain and depression) while following the course of treatment prescribed by your doctor.

If you have been living with hypothyroidism for some time, this book is for you, too. Thyroid hormone levels can fluctuate, even after several years of medication therapy, and require new treatment protocols. New ways to cope with lingering effects of hypothyroidism are constantly being developed and can, I hope, be of use to you. And a fresh perspective on your condition might introduce you to a more effective way of approaching nagging problems—and help you to overcome them.

Lastly, but not least, this book can serve as a learning tool for those who care for and about hypothyroid patients. Because a chronic illness affects not only the patient but also a patient's family members, friends, coworkers and even strangers sometimes, the more everyone becomes educated about the condition, its symptoms, and treatments, the better off everyone, especially the patient, will be.

In addition to systemic lupus erythematosus (SLE) and a host of other autoimmune disorders, I have Hashimoto's thyroiditis. In writing this book, I have called upon my own firsthand experience as well as the insights and suggestions of medical professionals and other thyroid patients. My approach is practical and positive: No matter how hopeless your life with hypothyroidism might seem, there are things you can do to improve your quality of life and help your body "turn the corner." Hypothyroidism is a chronic condition and requires regular, careful monitoring. But it is not a fatal illness and it need not stop you from achieving goals and making dreams come true, nor should it prevent you from taking control of your condition—and your life with it.

A diagnosis of hypothyroidism might seem like a marvelous gift at first. Like many patients, you might have experienced your symptoms for months or years before a physician finally identified what was causing them. Hearing your doctor tell you that you have an "underactive thyroid gland" and that your metabolism has slowed down because of it might make you feel in control for the first time in a long while.

Still you probably have a host of questions in your head and heart.

"How long will it take me to feel well again?"

"Will I ever be able to lose weight?"

"Does the medication I take cause side effects?"

"What causes hypothyroidism?"

"Will my children become hypothyroid?"

After your relief subsides, you also might be assailed by a confusing combination of emotions and a sense of helplessness at dealing with them effectively, at least right now. Feelings of relief at finally getting a diagnosis might give way to anger, frustration, confusion, and guilt. These are all natural for a person coping with a chronic illness. But that doesn't make them any easier to deal with.

In fact, hypothyroidism is perhaps the most frustrating and confusing health problem that plagues between six and seven million Americans, mostly women over the age of forty.[1] Although medication can help regulate the thyroid gland function and bring hormone production into the "normal" range with fairly predictable surety, the symptoms of living with an underactive thyroid gland are not so easily controlled. In fact, they often linger long after the underlying hormones are back in balance. And they can worsen if patients don't have their thyroid condition regularly and carefully monitored, or if they develop other illnesses or conditions and don't have those properly diagnosed and treated.

Especially in their early days of treatment, hypothyroid patients might live with only partially satisfying qualities of life. They may struggle with cosmetic deficiencies (hair loss, brittle nails, skin rashes), weight gain, fatigue, eye problems, and psychological effects, including depression, anxiety, and loss of self-worth. Quite often, an untreated or under-treated hypothyroid patient experiences a profound and debilitating fatigue. This affects the patient's productivity, enthusiasm for life, and, even, responsiveness to and eagerness for intimacy.

Acquiring knowledge about what is happening inside your body is crucial to being able to take charge of your health and emotional well-being and work successfully with your medical team. If you're reading this book, you have taken an important step toward improving your prognosis: You are making a positive move to give yourself the tools to make your life satisfying, even wonderful!

What happened to me

My journey into hypothyroidism has been a long and circuitous one. In 1982, after completing one rigorous year of graduate school, I thought my body was "short-circuiting." I was gaining weight, having trouble concentrating, and suffering from extreme fatigue, anxiety, and edginess (what a combination!). My usually comforting prayer life and faith didn't seem to take the edge off of my symptoms. I wasn't running a fever and didn't have signs of infection, but I still felt something was physically wrong.

That summer, I was working in Washington, D.C. It became more difficult for me to get through each day, and my moods became more mercurial. I asked a friend for a referral to a doctor and made an appointment.

Even as I described my symptoms, I thought I sounded like more of a complainer than someone with a health problem would.

"I'm gaining weight. I don't feel like going to work. I'm moody."

I could almost hear the violin in the background playing, "My heart cries for you . . ."

Thankfully, my doctor was a good listener. He ran a battery of tests, and I was hopeful that the mystery of my condition would be solved.

But everything, every test, came back in the normal range.

As I sat in his office going over the lab reports with him, I thought he was going to utter the dreaded words, "It's all in your head."

I'm going crazy, I remember thinking. *I'm making this all up.*

But instead of dismissing me, the doctor reached for his telephone.

"There's one test that hasn't come back yet," he said. "I'm sure it's all right, but I'll just call the lab . . ."

I said a silent prayer then, asking God for answers, any answers, to all my symptoms.

Moments later, my doctor's expression and manner changed completely. We had the answer.

My thyroid function was so high it was way off the scale!

At the time, I didn't know about TSH, T_3, T_4, or anything regarding the function of the thyroid gland. I didn't know that when the thyroid gland malfunctions, the whole body can be affected. However that day, I learned that my metabolism was so overactive that it was, in a sense, burning out the rest of my body.

My heart was overwhelmed with relief. My symptoms weren't all in my head. They were legitimate manifestations of a metabolism out of control.

I underwent more tests, including a thyroid uptake and scan, which confirmed that I had Graves' disease, an autoimmune condition that causes hyperactivity of the thyroid gland. There were three courses of treatment available to me: surgery (to remove part or all of the thyroid gland), medication, or treatment with radioactive iodine. I chose to take the medication, propythiouracil (PTU).

When I explained my condition to my mother, I learned that both of my grandmothers had had hyperactive thyroid glands. They had undergone surgery to have their glands removed and were put on synthetic thyroid hormone for the rest of their lives. Learning this was another source of relief: I wasn't alone! I had come by my Graves' disease honestly!

Even with my relief and excitement at being diagnosed, I knew that returning to graduate school was out of the question. I was still too symptomatic to undertake the extra stress of a difficult academic challenge. So I decided to work, instead, "waiting out" the time while my body readjusted.

It took a year and a half for my thyroid levels to fall back into the normal range. Gradually, I lost weight and felt calmer. I enrolled in a translation program and worked a more-than-full-time job. I traveled in Europe and the United States. After a few years, I re-enrolled in graduate school and this time was able to finish.

I continued to have my thyroid hormones monitored regularly and, on at least two occasions, had to go back on PTU because my levels and symptoms crept back up. But my symptoms never approached the horrendous levels of when I was first diagnosed with Graves'.

Then, in 1997, my health spiraled out of control once again. While working and traveling, I began to experience horrific symptoms of joint pain, feelings of choking, extreme fatigue, hair loss, and hearing loss. After a year of wondering what was wrong, I insisted my doctor do complete blood tests and was diagnosed with lupus.

In the early days of coping with lupus, I really did not think much about my thyroid function, although I continued to have it monitored. Three years after being diagnosed with lupus, my trusted endocrinologist died suddenly. His death was shocking to me—somehow I never expected that a doctor would die while still in the prime of life.

Partly because of my sadness at losing a trusted physician and partly out of convenience, I decided not to find another endocrinologist. Instead, I asked my rheumatologist to check my thyroid levels occasionally. One year later, I lost half of each of my eyebrows.

Because of lupus, I had already lost all the hair on my head. I had become accustomed to wearing wigs and hats (although I didn't like doing it). But the eyebrow loss was strange and difficult to conceal (they don't make wigs for eyebrows!). In addition, I noted that I was experiencing a kind of fatigue different from the lupus variety (which is bone-numbing and all-encompassing). I felt lethargic, heavy, as though there was just not enough "gas in the tank." I had difficulty concentrating and remembering things. I was always losing my keys, checkbook, address list . . .

Besides lupus, I had developed Sjogren's syndrome, vasculitis, and a host of new symptoms and problems. I wasn't eager to add another illness to the list, but I had kept up with prayer and meditation. I listened closely to my body and to God's presence in my life. And I decided that I should have my thyroid more closely examined.

After asking my rheumatologist for a referral to an endocrinologist, I went for a complete endocrine exam. My new doctor ascertained that my overactive thyroid had "gone full circle" and was now underactive: From Graves' disease, I'd gone to Hashimoto's thyroiditis.

Once again, my symptoms, including the odd eyebrow loss and inexplicable weight gain, made thyroid sense. I threw myself into finding out as much as I could about this new condition. I learned about TSH, T_3, T_4, the body's metabolic and hormonal system, and the implications of this new diagnosis for my total health picture. I also learned about the research that is being conducted (finally!) and the possibilities for better understanding and treatment of this so-called "woman's disease." And I learned about the community of fellow hypothyroid sufferers, men and women who are remarkable, resilient, and full of positive suggestions and anecdotes to inspire and enlighten hypothyroid "newbies."

My thyroid education served to allay my fears about my future living with Hashimoto's thyroiditis. It also helped me take control of another area of my health, a very positive thing, and brought me renewed faith and hope that there are answers to even the most confounding problems.

Why I wrote this book

When I was diagnosed with Hashimoto's thyroiditis, I immediately found that much of the available information was outdated, incomplete, or scattered across many different publications and Web sites. Although I thrive in doing research, I began to wonder if there wouldn't be a value in putting vital information concerning hypothyroidism in one, easy-to-use volume. It is often very difficult to conduct a full-on Internet search when you're too tired to sit up in a chair!

As I learned more about my condition, I further discovered that much of the available suggestions for treatment were impractical, controversial, or incompatible with my approach to my healthcare. In addition, many of the sources were biased against the very treatments that my doctors advocated, and I sensed that these proponents of more alternative therapies were perhaps giving advice inconsistent with my experience and medically unsound.

I tend to be realistic and positive about treatments suggested by my doctors and cautious of promises of "quick cures" from alternative venues. I recognize that alternative therapies hold much promise, and some can assist hypothyroid patients to cope better with their symptoms. Still, I am "Western medicine friendly," meaning that I believe that most physicians, particularly specialists such as rheumatologists and endocrinologists, are eager to help their patients improve their wellness to the full extent of their expertise. Responsible doctors also operate within the boundaries of the healthcare system, guidelines for diagnosing patients and prescribing medications, and the professional standards of their chosen vocation. They are as human as you or me, but they possess a body of knowledge and experience that, coupled with their willingness to assist their patients, make them essential resources for our definitive healthcare.

Another philosophy of mine greatly influences this book. I believe that we patients hold tremendous responsibility for the quality and effectiveness of our healthcare. We did not cause our illnesses. But there are things we have control over. We choose whom we go to for treatment, and we decide how disciplined and consistent we will be in following through with our appointments and treatments. We also decide the amount and type of information we allow to influence us in working with our physicians. By working together, patient and physician can forge a nurturing, healing relationship that will hold both in good stead. I believe strongly in quality healthcare being a "two-way street."

I wrote this book to assemble high-quality, up-to-date information about hypothyroidism and to put it all together in one patient-friendly volume. Although we share the same disorder, our health "pictures" are unique. Some of us have multiple autoimmune diseases, and others only have hypothyroidism. I hope that this book will serve you well to grasp the basics about hypothyroidism and provide details that will illuminate your individual situation.

How to use this book

The format of this book is unlike any other volume dealing with hypothyroidism because it takes a chronological approach, from the day you are diagnosed through the entire first year of living with the condition. I know well that there is a lot to learn, but also that there are a lot of emotions that you will need to work through to be able to take charge of your life with hypothyroidism. By taking a day-by-day approach, you will be able to assimilate information in manageable pieces. If you were diagnosed a while ago, I still encourage you to start with Day 1 and go through the book chronologically, at your own pace.

You will notice that there are no chapters in this book. Instead, there are Days, Weeks, and Months. Each is divided into a Living and a Learning section. In the Living sections, you will find information and insight into emotionally, spiritually, and personally coping with hypothyroidism. I have spoken with fellow hypothyroid patients, and their comments and suggestions are included in these sections, too. Hearing from a range of people living with the same thing you are will help you understand even more fully that you are not alone—there are many other people who are hypothyroid, too, and they want to help you be strong, proactive, and positive.

The Learning sections contain information and interviews about specific topics pertaining to the medicine and science of hypothyroidism. These include a brief history of thyroid science, and the basics about the thyroid gland, the endocrine system, and how it all ties in with your metabolism, symptoms, and course of treatment. I'll introduce you to the different medical professionals and organizations that can give you treatment and support as you continue in your life with hypothyroidism, and I'll talk about the tests that you might need to have and the different kinds of medication that are available at this time.

The more you learn about what's going on inside your body, the better off you'll be, but don't be daunted by the technical aspects of these sections. My aim is not to intimidate you, but rather to give you the basics so that you can have informed conversations with your doctor and come to a good, solid understanding of how to live well with hypothyroidism. Sidebars provide you with important material, too, and the words in **boldface** are defined in a glossary at the back of this book.

I will not prescribe

I am not a doctor and I will not prescribe for you. Moreover, I will not tell you what treatments you should follow, nor will I recommend dosages of medications or combinations of vitamins, drugs, or herbs. Your health history and current condition are unique to you, and there is no one-size-fits-all protocol for treating your total wellness. Also, research into the treatments and causes of hypothyroidism is ongoing, and the protocols used today might be obsolete tomorrow. For these reasons, you should rely on your physician to guide you in what is best for you at any particular time and for any particular health issue.

The symptoms associated with hypothyroidism can be many and varied, and I discuss them in this book. Do not assume that you will experience all of them, nor worry that your present symptoms will worsen to the extreme. Your symptoms are individual to you, and their degree of severity is also unique.

Sometimes, I will share my own or others' experiences with medications or approaches to the symptoms from hypothyroidism, but, again, I am not recommending these to you. Every aspect of your health, including what medications you take or what other paths of treatment you wish to explore, should be discussed with your personal doctor. Only he or she has the qualifications and perspective to give you informed, specific diagnoses and guidance.

Where the focus is

This book is for people who are living through their first year after being diagnosed with hypothyroidism. Although I discuss some of the symptoms of hypothyroidism, I do not mean for this book to be used as a diagnostic tool for those who do not yet have definitive word from their physicians that they are hypothyroid. My discussion of symptoms is for the purpose of articulating some of the issues already-diagnosed patients have to cope with as they commence their course of treatment. It is also to serve as a refresher for patients who are wondering if their thyroid replacement therapy needs to be modified.

Through my own experience and in speaking with others who live with hypothyroidism, I have learned that the best focus is one that is centered on healthy, nurturing living and responsibility. The information included in this book is meant to be a positive means to gain knowledge and resolve to meet your challenges head-on. You won't find a "pity party" here, but I hope you will find reason to celebrate your renewed resolve and thrive in your life with hypothyroidism.

Another tool that I've found essential to finding and maintaining balance in my life is to keep all aspects of it as effectively simple as possible. This holds true to my approach to health, also, and I've tried to convey this in this book. Instead of piling on the treatments, for example, I have found that taking each additional therapy one step and one dose at a time helps to lessen the stress of trying something new. It also enables me and my healthcare givers to determine just how effective each new treatment or medication is and to make necessary adjustments accordingly. Keeping my approach to finding information simple helps me to gain a firm knowledge base, which serves me well when learning about new treatments and protocols. So, I've consulted with the "tried and true" sources, first: thyroid associations, medical texts and teaching institutions, and patients who've successfully lived with hypothyroidism for a long time. Added to this base of knowledge, then, is information from alternative sources and news reports of cutting-edge research and therapies. The result is a well-rounded body of information, giving a practical, effective perspective on which to base a healthful approach to coping with hypothyroidism.

Keep on learning

Living with hypothyroidism is a long-term proposition. After the first year following your diagnosis, you will need to monitor your thyroid hormone levels, follow your prescribed course of treatment, and keep on learning about new developments in endocrinology and healthcare in general. Many patients rely upon their doctors for insight into new methods of coping with their medical conditions. There is nothing wrong with this, but there is nothing wrong, too, with taking news reports or information about the latest research or treatments to your doctor and discussing them with him or her. The more informed you are, the better off your prognosis will be.

There are many ways to continue learning about hypothyroidism. Using this book as a guide, you can refresh your knowledge of the basics of thyroid function and apply that information to your progress. As a further jumping-off point, I list a number of thyroid-related organizations and books for your information. I encourage you to explore what they have to offer both in terms of patient services and continued education.

The Internet is a valuable resource for up-to-the-minute medical news as well as access to the thyroid community throughout the world. I have provided you with some jumping-off points. You will, no doubt, find many more Web sources. You will need to be careful about what information you take as truth; there is much solid data, but also much fluff online. I've included some tips about sifting through what you will find on the Internet, as well as two Web sites that are dedicated to shedding light and finding the truth in "Web-disseminated urban legends," which periodically find their way into our email boxes.

The personal testimonies of other hypothyroid patients are terrific sources of inspiration, as well as of new information. In this book, I have included parts of conversations with other patients (I have changed their names to protect their privacy). In fact, each year, thousands of people in the United States are diagnosed with hypothyroidism. This means that thousands of people are just learning about their test results, just realizing that they have a chronic illness, just beginning to go through the emotional, spiritual, and physical journey that you are embarking upon now. As you continue to live with hypothyroidism and discover what treatments and lifestyle modifications work for you, I encourage you to share your learning with others. In doing so, you will be helping to build our hypothyroid community into a strong, resilient, hopeful, supportive group. You are not alone. We're with one another each step, each day, all along the way.

THE FIRST YEAR™

Hypothyroidism

What a Relief!

YOUR DOCTOR has confirmed that you are hypo-thyroid—at last! The first thing you feel is quite possibly a sense of profound, almost giddy relief. I know that feeling—I had exactly that reaction when I was diagnosed with Hashimoto's thyroiditis, an **autoimmune** condition that causes the thyroid gland to shut down.

Some people might think it strange to feel relief at being diagnosed with a medical problem. Don't worry. You are really reacting quite naturally. The symptoms of hypothyroidism can be so non-specific that doctors often dismiss them when patients first present themselves. Like many other hypothyroid patients, you might have gone weeks, months, even years with-out a diagnosis. Your symptoms might have become very acute, and you might have even despaired that you would ever feel well again.

No wonder you are relieved when your doctor tells you your thyroid is hypoactive!

Looking back over the long road

Julie N. began to experience symptoms during the summer after the birth of her second child, but was not diagnosed until almost two years later. "I was feeling lethargic, not losing weight very fast, and feeling somewhat unwell, in an unspecified sort of way. I had lost some hair during my pregnancy, and the bald spot did not grow back. There was swelling in my knees, too."

Over the next few months, her symptoms changed drastically, and she became hyperactive.

"My body was racing at a very high level and I could get no rest. I was also losing weight. In addition, I blushed easily—this was unusual for me— and felt very unsure of myself. By December 1978, I was becoming dangerously psychotic."

After going to a psychiatrist, who prescribed sleeping pills but did not do a physical exam, Julie went to her family physician. He did a series of blood tests and found that her thyroid function had completely shut down.

"He told me, given the evidence of the blood tests, I should not have been able to stand up. It was a great relief to discover that I was not going crazy and that I had an understandable physical condition that could be treated."

Because it can take a long time to get the proper diagnosis and start on treatment, another natural reaction to the diagnosis is one of anger.

"My hair was falling out. I had super dry skin. My heels cracked. I could never get warm. My periods were real bad, and I had awful PMS, too. It went on for a while. It was horrible," said Pamela G. "I had a doctor that I went to all the time. He diagnosed me as borderline hypothyroid and told me to call him in six weeks if I wasn't better. I pitched a horrific fit."

On this first day of the rest of your life living with hypothyroidism, accept your relief as a natural reaction to waiting so long for a diagnosis. Also, acknowledge your anger. In this day of modern diagnostic tools and highly trained medical professionals, it is frustrating, sometimes even outrageous, that someone in physical distress should have to wait a long time for a diagnosis of hypothyroidism. But don't let your relief lull you into a sense that your health is no longer an issue in your life, and don't let anger eat away at you. Use both these emotions as productive means to take the first steps toward treating and controlling your health.

A *positive from a negative*

Both your relief and your anger can help you in the days, weeks, and months ahead as you begin to take control of your health. Relief can give you the enthusiasm and focus you need to make sense of the medication regime your doctor may prescribe, as well as to inspire you to look at all the aspects of your life that have been affected by your underactive thyroid—and do something about them.

Anger can be a tricky emotion. On the one hand, you could be justified in being angry with your doctors for not diagnosing you sooner. However, if you let anger take hold of you, it can prevent you from placing trust in the very people upon whom you have to rely for guidance in treating your condition.

The best thing to do when you are angry is to acknowledge your emotion, but act in your best interest to proceed with the treatment that your physician feels is best at this time.

If you disagree with your doctor's prescribed course of treatment, or feel that he or she is not fully qualified to handle a thyroid problem, consult with a reputable **endocrinologist**. Make sure that he or she focuses on thyroid (some endocrinologists prefer to focus on diabetes or other aspects of their specialty). Explain to your other doctor that you wish to get a second opinion and ask for copies of your medical files, including test results. Usually, this is not a problem, especially if you approach your doctor professionally. Again, acknowledge that you are angry, but act only in ways that will enable you to get the best possible care.

Take a deep breath

The day that you receive your diagnosis can be completely overwhelming. Besides coping with your many emotions, you have a lot to learn, including how to take your medication and what effects your condition has had—and will have—on your whole life. Sometime during that first day, take some quiet time to allow yourself to breathe, to reflect upon the new turn your life has taken. Relax into your relief and out of your feelings of frustration and anger. Pray or meditate on strength for the days ahead and on gratitude for finally getting answers to your questions.

Above all, approach the world of hypothyroidism in manageable pieces. Take one step, one day at a time and you will find and embrace remarkable things all along the way.

IN A SENTENCE:

> *Being diagnosed with hypothyroidism means your long, hard road of wondering what's wrong with you is finally over.*

learning

What Is Hypothyroidism?

THE THYROID gland is butterfly-shaped and is located at the front of your neck. Its two "wings" are called lobes and the middle section is called the isthmus. It is part of the **endocrine** system, an internal collection of hormone-secreting glands, and produces hormones that are essential for the proper functioning of your metabolism, the rate at which each organ in your body functions. When the thyroid gland is working properly, your body's metabolism is in balance. When it malfunctions, your whole body can be affected.

Two kinds of malfunction

When the thyroid gland is producing an overabundance of hormone (**hyperthyroidism**), your body can go into overdrive, causing heart palpitations, weight loss, sleeplessness, and a host of other symptoms.

When your thyroid gland is underactive, you have a condition called hypothyroidism, and your body slows down…sometimes *way* down. You might become emotionally as well as physically listless, even depressed. Your appearance might change radically in the form of weight gain and skin and hair problems. You might feel like you have a lingering illness, akin to the flu, and have exacerbation of asthma or allergic reactions.

SOME of the symptoms of hypothyroidism include:

Dull, persistent fatigue

Slow heartbeat

Skin rashes

Muscular weakness and stiffness

Weight gain (usually not more than 10 lbs.)

Constipation

Swelling and puffiness

Menstrual irregularities (especially heavy periods, sometimes clotting)

Depression

Forgetfulness

Difficulty concentrating

Hair loss (especially the lateral eye brows)

Goiter (enlargement of the thyroid gland)

At first, you might take your symptoms as only the effects of living in a hectic world. But as you now know, there is an internal reason for how you feel.

The most common reason for thyroid failure in the United States is that of autoimmune destruction of the thyroid, called Hashimoto's thyroiditis. There are several other reasons why the thyroid gland slows down and/or stops producing its metabolic hormones. In some parts of the world, lack of iodine in the diet results in inadequate thyroid hormone production. Other times, removing all or part of the thyroid gland because it is overactive or, in rare cases, cancerous, results in a hypothyroid condition. Sometimes, babies are born with thyroid abnormalities, which is quite serious and can lead to **cretinism** if left untreated. For this reason, every newborn should have his or her thyroid checked to make sure it is functioning normally. Another reason for loss of thyroid function is exposure to radiation in high doses. Many people who lived near the Chernobyl nuclear plant in the then-Soviet Union when it suffered a meltdown, as well as others who were in the path of the cloud of the resulting radiation, contracted thyroid cancer and lost thyroid function.

Because the hypothalamus-pituitary-thyroid axis is so sensitive to each of these glands' functions, any problem with one of them might cause problems for all three. So, although it is very rare, it is important that your doctor rule out any hypothalamus or pituitary problems when he or she is checking your thyroid. This is just a precaution; usually low thyroid hormone production is due to a problem with the thyroid gland. But it is always better to be absolutely sure.

The number of people in the United States who suffer from inadequate iodine is very small because there is significant iodine in salt and other food products. According to the Thyroid Cancer Survivors Association, Inc. (ThyCa), thyroid cancer is the most common endocrine cancer. The American Cancer Society estimates that 20,700 new cases of thyroid cancer will be diagnosed in 2002.[2]

Hashimoto's thyroiditis

Hashimoto's thyroiditis is named after Hakaru Hashimoto, a Japanese doctor who first described the condition in 1912.[3] Before that time, thyroid underactivity had been documented by doctors and even treated by feeding the patient a serum containing sheep's thyroid. However, Hashimoto was the first to determine the condition subsequently found to be autoimmune in nature.

An autoimmune condition is one in which the body produces **antibodies** or **T lymphocytes** (types of white blood cells active in the immune process) against a person's own body tissue. So, instead of fighting off a virus or allergen from the outside, the autoimmune antibodies attack an organ or organs within the body.

In Graves' disease, the antibodies clearly produce the disease. In Hashimoto's thyroiditis, it is unknown whether the antibodies or T cells (lymphocytes) damage the gland. It is thought that when the antibodies become active, the thyroid gland's function is compromised and begins to slow down. Often, over time, the thyroid gland stops functioning altogether. Usually, this condition cannot be reversed, however it can be treated with replacement thyroid hormone so that a patient's metabolism continues to function comfortably.

Many people possess the antibodies to the thyroid gland, however most will never become symptomatic and will not need treatment. According to Basil Rapoport, M.B., a research **thyroidologist**, approximately 10 percent of patients with antibodies against the thyroid gland will become hypothyroid. The ratio of women to men with hypothyroidism is approximately 5:1 or 6:1.

Not much is known about what triggers the antibodies to begin attacking the thyroid gland. It could even be that the antibodies that can be easily measured are only markers of the condition, not the antibodies that actually cause the condition. There is some evidence that there could be a genetic propensity toward autoimmune disease; however, a parent with Hashimoto's thyroiditis will not necessarily pass it along to his or her children. Also, because so many people can have thyroid antibodies without ever becoming symptomatic, researchers believe that there are also environmental factors that contribute to "turning on" the autoimmune process. Some theories are that stressful events, infection, certain chemicals, smoke, pollution, and other substances might play a role in beginning the autoimmune process.

Research into the complexities of the autoimmune process is ongoing, and someday we will know much more about why particular people become symptomatic while others do not. For now, it is important to know that although your hypothyroidism cannot be cured, it can be treated.

Hyperthyroidism and hypothyroidism

In some cases, it is possible to start off with a hyperactive thyroid and end up hypoactive. This happened to me. For almost twenty years, I lived with Graves' disease, an autoimmune condition that causes the thyroid gland to be hyperactive. Then, suddenly, my metabolism slowed down. It really felt as though someone hit the brakes and I came screeching to a halt!

When I was diagnosed with Graves' disease, my doctor told me that in some cases, the thyroid gland eventually burns itself out and hyperthyroid patients become hypothyroid. After researching this a bit further, I learned that there was more than just coincidence to this statement.

The same phenomenon that causes Graves' disease also causes Hashimoto's thyroiditis. That is, the body produces antibodies that attack the thyroid gland. Whether these antibodies produce a hyperthyroid condition or a hypothyroid one is unpredictable. However, once thyroid antibodies are present, they do not go away. Many times, patients have both antibodies and what happens is that they can reverse their earlier course and cause the opposite condition to occur.

"Graves' disease and Hashimoto's really stem from the same thing," says Dr. Rapoport. "A person who is hyperthyroid can become hypothyroid. Sometimes, too, that person can swing back and forth for a time."

Usually, however, the thyroid gland does "burn itself out" over time.

Thyroid cancer

In some cases, the thyroid gland might develop one or more lumps. Very often, these lumps are benign (non-cancerous) nodes caused by multinodular goiter often found in Hashimoto's thyroiditis. This can be diagnosed through fine-needle aspiration biopsy, where the doctor inserts a needle into the node, draws out the fluid it contains, then analyzes it in a laboratory. Though it is rare, the thyroid lumps could be cancerous and need to be treated more radically.

Just as with autoimmune thyroid problems, there is some evidence that many thyroid cancers are, in part, caused by a genetic predisposition to them. Other times, exposure to high doses of radiation might trigger the development of lumps in the thyroid gland that become cancerous. Thankfully, in most cases thyroid cancer is very treatable. Also, it is usually slow-growing and seldom spreads beyond the thyroid gland. Treatments for thyroid cancer can include removal of part or all of the gland, chemotherapy, and/or radiation therapy. Usually, patients who have undergone treatment for thyroid cancer must take supplemental thyroid hormone to make up for what has been lost due to radiation and/or surgical treatments.

Exposure to excess radiation

Patients who suffer thyroid cancer due to excessive radiation exposure tend to have a more aggressive form of the disease than others, as was seen in patients who were affected by the nuclear accident at Chernobyl in the former Soviet Union. This is because the thyroid gland absorbs radioactive iodine, and most nuclear explosions or accidents involving nuclear power plants release it. The result is severe damage to the gland and development of malignant growths or tumors.[4] Exposure to routine radiation sources, such as mammograms or other X rays and treatment of Graves' disease with radioactive iodine, should not bring about the kind of extensive thyroid damage that has been seen at places such as those around Chernobyl.

Men who are hypothyroid

Although the majority of people with hypothyroidism are women, men can also suffer from the condition. Their symptoms are usually similar to those seen in women, although the way they approach treatment might be different. For example, women might be more willing than men to seek psychological help for emotional problems.

The medicines used to treat hypothyroidism in men are the same as those given to women. Dosages and combinations of hormones are determined by doctors using the same normal ranges in tests as for women, and the follow-up is also identical.

Hypothyroidism in children and teenagers

A small number of young people will develop hypothyroidism each year. They might show no symptoms at all, or they might experience growth problems, difficulties in developing their sexuality (including delays in menstruation and breast development), and cognitive dysfunction. Because the growth process is so crucial to overall good health, children or teens who are hypothyroid need expert medical attention and encouragement as they go through thyroid treatment and learn to manage their disorder.

IN A SENTENCE:

> *Hypothyroidism is a condition where your thyroid gland becomes underactive, causing your metabolism to slow down.*

DAY 2

living

Why Me?

AFTER FEELING the initial "whoosh" of relief that you have a firm diagnosis of hypothyroidism, you will undoubtedly find yourself wondering why you ever developed the condition in the first place. You might ask yourself if you did anything to bring it about. Or you might hear stories about supposed causes of hypothyroidism that lead you to believe that you made yourself sick.

You might begin to feel very guilty.

Your parents, too, might be overwhelmed with guilt, thinking they gave you the genes or did something else to cause you to become hypothyroid. Perhaps your diagnosis ignited a family squabble. You might have heard one of your parents exclaim to the other, "She got it from *your* side!"

It's not your fault

Although there could be environmental factors, coupled with genetic propensities, linked to developing autoimmune hypothyroidism, there is no proof that a person can bring on hypothyroidism him- or herself. The endocrine system is complex and reacts to so many influences that your actions cannot tip the scale one way or the other.

Know this for certain: You are not to blame for your medical condition.

Likewise, even though one or both of the branches of your family to whom you are directly linked might carry some genes associated with auto-immune illness, this does not guarantee that you or any of your other relatives will come down with hypothyroidism or any other disease. In my case, for example, both of my grandmothers were hyperthyroid. But of the other members of my family, only I have had any thyroid problems (at least, so far).

Of course, it helps to know what your family's medical history is. There could be a greater likelihood for someone to develop thyroid problems if a family member already has them. But no parent or other relative should feel guilty that he or she "gave you" thyroid disease. This simply does not happen.

Denial

My friends who have one or more chronic illnesses and I have a saying that we use whenever we think one of us is inching toward denial. It's, "Ah, you've decided to take a long trip down that river in Egypt, have you?"

What river?

That "old river of denial."

Even if you accept your hypothyroidism completely, you are likely to slip into denial at some point in the future. Perhaps you will feel so good after medication therapy that you'll think you don't need to take pills anymore. Or your thyroid levels will be in the normal range long enough for you to think that you're fine. If you still have trouble losing weight, or if your hair doesn't grow back even after you have been on your medication a while, you might doubt that hypothyroidism is your problem after all.

Or if you've been healthy all your life, it could be very hard for you to accept that you now have a chronic illness. You might not want to believe that you are ill because you'd never "do that to yourself" (going back to the feelings of guilt that can sometimes arise). If a trusted loved one thinks the doctor might have made a mistake, maybe you pick up on this and take it to heart.

Maybe my loved one is right, and the doctor is wrong, you might think.

If you have been told by your doctor that you are "borderline" hypothyroid, you might deny that you could ever go over the edge into full-blown hypothyroidism. This denial might prevent you from taking care of yourself properly and monitoring the situation. Although it might comfort you at the moment, in the long run, it can be dangerous.

Indeed, falling into denial can make you ignore your health. It can cause you to do things that are actually *bad* for you and exacerbate your symptoms. For example, if you do not believe that you are hypothyroid, you might take over-the-counter medications that are contraindicated for you and do yourself harm.

Left untreated for a long period of time, hypothyroidism can bring your whole body to such a state that you might become psychotic or fall apart physically. If this happens, it will take much longer for you to put yourself back together again, and you might find that you have done permanent damage to, for example, your heart.

Is there any good that comes from being in denial?

Perhaps.

Some denial might be beneficial, because it allows you to digest your health situation in manageable pieces. You might be completely overwhelmed if you had to learn everything about hypothyroidism all at once. Denial can help you gradually move into full awareness of your illness and what you have to do to take care of yourself. But you need to understand that eventually, you will have to accept your condition and take steps to help yourself feel better.

Coping with denial

If you know yourself very well, you can probably gauge when your sense of denial is working against your own good. Friends are also excellent barometers of if or how deeply you are falling into denial. They can be your sounding board for when you have doubts, or your critics when you seem to be glossing over or ignoring things that are important. Your doctor, too, can help you deal with your denial. He or she can emphasize the analysis of your exam and test results and can also impress upon you the importance of taking your medication in the prescribed dosages.

Make use of your support system and medical team early on and throughout your treatment to ensure that if you do take the "trip down that river in Egypt" you will not linger but will arrive at your destination—acceptance—in a healthful, responsible way.

Depression

Perhaps one of the symptoms you have been experiencing since you started to feel unwell is depression. This is a common complaint, particularly for those who suffer from hypothyroidism. There are psychological reasons for this, but there are concrete medical reasons, too. It is very important that you are able to communicate clearly and openly with your doctor so that all the threads of your depression can lead you to the proper balance of medical and psychological help.

Signs of depression

In its mildest form, depression causes you to feel like you have the "blues." You don't enjoy leisure activities as much as you once did, and you also don't find a lot of pleasure in beloved relationships. It's harder for you to get out of bed in the morning, and when you do engage in activity, you feel disconnected from what's going on around you.

More severe cases of depression can manifest themselves in psychotic episodes, where someone becomes delusional or has other extreme emotional outbursts. Remember Julie N.? She went so long without a diagnosis that she called a psychiatrist because she was afraid she might hurt herself or someone else.

Fortunately, in many cases depression abates as a hypothyroid patient begins and continues treatment. Getting through the time between when you begin feeling depressed and when your medication "kicks in" can be a challenge, but it is possible. And the more you understand about what's going on inside your body and accept that your emotional swings are not "all in your head," the more prepared you will be to cope with your emotions in a positive, nurturing way.

IN A SENTENCE:

You are not to blame for becoming hypothyroid.

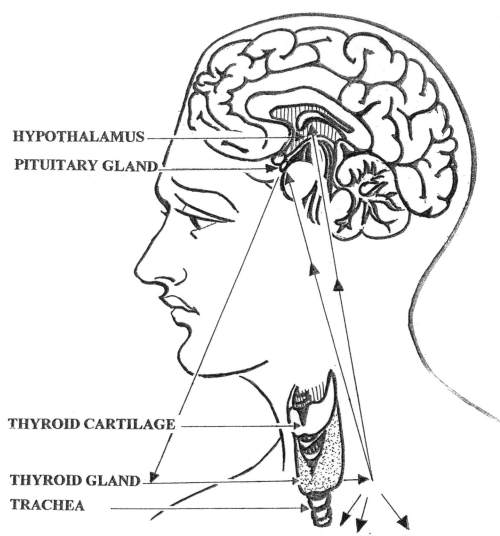

HYPOTHALAMUS

PITUITARY GLAND

THYROID CARTILAGE

THYROID GLAND

TRACHEA

THE HYPOTHALAMUS SECRETES TRH (THYROTROPIN-RELEASING HORMONE), WHICH GOES TO THE PITUITARY GLAND. THE PITUITARY GLAND THEN SECRETES TSH (THYROID-STIMULATING HORMONE), WHICH TRAVELS TO THE THYROID GLAND, WHICH PRODUCES T4 AND T3. THESE TRAVEL THROUGHOUT THE BODY INCLUDING THE HYPOTHALAMUS AND THE PITUITARY GLAND.

Illustration by Donal Keohane

learning

All about the Hormones

THE ESSENTIAL function of the thyroid gland is to produce **hormones**. Hormones are organic (natural) substances that have specific effects upon other areas of the body. Thyroid hormones affect all aspects of your **metabolism**, which is the rate at which your organs and bodily functions operate. The thyroid gland secretes two hormones: levothyroxine (T_4) and L-triiodothyronine (T_3). The hormone that is most active in physiologic terms is T_3, but other hormones also play a part in the cycle that has such a significant effect upon metabolism.

A hormone-driven cycle

Fueling thyroid hormone production begins with a gland called the **hypothalamus.** It releases thyrotropin-releasing hormone (TRH), which travels to the anterior **pituitary**, where it stimulates secretion of thyrotropin stimulating hormone (TSH). TSH, in turn, stimulates the thyroid gland to produce T_4 and about 20 percent of the body's supply of T_3. The other 80 percent of T_3 is derived from T_4 when that hormone is deiodonized, or converted, in peripheral tissues.

In most cases of hypothyroidism, the thyroid gland doesn't produce enough T_4 and/or T_3 and the pituitary increases its production of TSH in order to stimulate the thyroid gland to produce more. In some rare cases, the pituitary slows down on its own. Accurate measurement of thyroid-related hormone levels could pinpoint just where the problem is.

How are hormones measured?

The easiest way to measure thyroid hormone levels is by having blood drawn and then sending it to a lab for study. Usually one vial of blood is enough to conduct all the tests needed to tell what is happening with your thyroid system. Sometimes it takes as long as one week to get the results back on your blood tests.

When you get your results back, you will see that the lab has assigned a numeric value to each of your thyroid levels. This correlates to a certain standard range of "normal," which can vary slightly from lab to lab. If your numerical results fall somewhere within that range, they are considered normal *for that range*. If they are lower or higher than the range, they are either "high" or "low."

Hormone levels are correlated to the lab's normal range. But that doesn't mean that what is normal according to the lab isn't below or above normal for you. Many people are told they are "borderline" hyper- or hypothyroid because their results fall in the lower or upper range of normal. These people might feel fine, or have some symptoms. Others function well at a certain level within normal, but feel unwell if their levels fluctuate, even within the "normal" numbers.

There is an ongoing debate among practitioners in the endocrinology community over what should be the proper ranges for hormone measurement. Some doctors believe that the current lab standards are not fine-tuned enough to reflect the true condition of many patients, especially for TSH. Other doctors believe that the current standards are just fine and have no intention of changing. If your thyroid hormone numbers are in your doctor's "normal" range and you still feel symptoms, discuss this with your doctor, but don't insist that he or she raise your medication levels. Perhaps your symptoms are due to other things besides thyroid disease and you need to explore this further.

AS a hypothyroid patient, you will probably have to have your blood drawn at regular intervals for the rest of your life. Here are some tips for making the experience less painful:

○ Take a deep breath just as the needle is inserted into your skin.

○ Don't look at the vial as it fills, and don't hold your breath, either.

○ Try to relax and focus on a pleasant thought or favorite song.

○ If you have thin veins or extremely sensitive skin, ask the phlebotomist (the person drawing your blood) to use a "butterfly," which is a thinner needle attached to a thin, long tube that carries the blood to the vial. A butterfly is often much easier on your skin and veins.

○ You can alleviate developing a bruise after giving blood by putting pressure on the puncture for 1–2 minutes after the phlebotomist has withdrawn the needle. Elevating your arm after you've given blood so that the puncture is above you heart and keeping it there for one minute might help, too.

Which hormones should be measured?

The American Association of Clinical Endocrinologists (AACE) suggests that the "most valuable test is a sensitive measure of TSH level," when establishing the diagnosis of hypothyroidism.[1] Some doctors rely on this test exclusively when diagnosing and monitoring patients with hypothyroid conditions. Other doctors test total T_4, T_3 resin uptake, and free T_4 to get a more comprehensive picture of what could be happening to thyroid hormone within your body. This information could, in turn, influence the amount or type of medication you will be given.

Another test is one for thyroid autoantibodies. These are positive in 95 percent of patients with Hashimoto's thyroiditis, and the presence of these antibodies are of great help in diagnosing this autoimmune condition. Once you have been tested for thyroid autoantibodies, it is usually unnecessary to be retested; although the levels can fluctuate, once they are present, they rarely disappear.

Special considerations for pregnancy

If you are hypothyroid and plan to become or are pregnant, you need to make sure that each of your attending physicians knows of your thyroid condition, as well as what medications you are taking and in what doses. Careful monitoring of your thyroid levels is important, particularly during the first trimester, when T_4 crosses the placenta in "substantial amounts," according to the AACE.[2] Thyroid imbalances in your unborn baby can cause impaired development, so by testing your thyroid, you are not just taking care of yourself, but your child, as well. In particular, finding out the levels of your TSH can help you and your doctor make better decisions about the types and amounts of any thyroid medications you might take during your pregnancy. In addition, there is some correlation between thyroperoxidase antibodies TPO-Ab levels in the first trimester and postpartum hypothyroidism and postpartum depression.[3]

Although the link is still under study, Dr. Rapoport says, "One-third of the women who have TPO-Ab during their first trimester are more likely to have postpartum depression." Testing for these antibodies can help you, your family, and your doctor better prepare for the days and months after you give birth.

The AACE has issued recommended guidelines for physicians who care for pregnant women. It is a good idea to be aware of these guidelines if you are now, or are thinking of becoming, pregnant and I have included some of the information that they recommend. Complete and current guidelines may be obtained from the AACE (www.aace.org).

The opposite of hyperthyroid

If you are like me and started out with Graves' disease, becoming hypothyroid can be a shock. With active Graves', you had energy, sometimes too much energy, and probably had no problem losing weight, or at least keeping the pounds from adding on. With hypothyroidism, you are tired, possibly depressed, and having difficulty keeping your weight under control.

The swing of hormones might also cause you to doubt yourself and the validity of your emotions. Are you *really* depressed, or is it your thyroid? Were you *really* happy when you were hyperthyroid, or was it just your hormones?

Becoming hypothyroid means you have to get to know yourself and your body all over again in some ways. But in other ways, you haven't changed at all.

As you adjust from being hyper- to hypo-, be kind to yourself. Understand that you will experience mood swings, that you have to change your lifestyle and way of thinking about your body in light of your new diagnosis. Above all, don't despair! You can be strong through it all, and experience good health as you learn how to take care of yourself in the best way possible.

IN A SENTENCE:

> *Thyroid hormones regulate the body's metabolism and testing them helps your doctor determine your diagnosis and course of treatment.*

living

Telling Others

WHEN YOU first get the diagnosis that you are hypothyroid, your relief might lead you to tell your friends, family, and coworkers. Of course, it is your right not to tell everyone, too; your health condition is your own business and you are entitled to your privacy in matters concerning it.

If you do choose to tell other people, however, although you are relieved, even giddy, about the news, others' reactions to it might not be so enthusiastic. This is due to several factors, among them the fact that not everyone understands what you've been going through and how significant it is that you finally have a firm diagnosis. Also, if your health has negatively impacted your job or relationships with others, chances are it will not be easy to erase the hurt or resentment that has built up. So, although you may *want* to tell everyone that you now know what was causing your symptoms, consider each relationship and each situation carefully and individually.

Turning to family

The people you rely upon most for support and encouragement throughout your illness are the people closest to you. Usually, these are your family members: parents, children, grandparents, aunts, uncles, cousins, and spouse. They are the people with whom you share life's most important moments, such as births, marriages, and religious rites. They are also the people with whom you share life's "smaller" moments—the artwork done by your toddler, the frustration at having a hectic schedule, the joke that you heard around the water cooler at work. It is no surprise, then, that you tell your family members first when you receive your diagnosis of hypothyroidism.

In the ideal world, if you tell a family member you have a chronic illness, they will respond by offering their unconditional love, support, and encouragement. Many families are tremendously supportive of their loved ones, especially if someone falls ill and needs extra attention and emotional, financial, or physical help.

You might be one of the very fortunate, blessed people whose family rallies around you when you receive your diagnosis. If so, treasure your loved ones even more than you did before. Be a friend to them as much as they are to you, and relax in their love and comfort. Share your triumphs with your family as you take charge of your symptoms and treatment and enjoy your presence among good, strong loved ones. And if you run into conflict concerning your diagnosis or condition, take each person, each reaction, one at a time.

Making sense of the troubled reactions

For many different reasons, even though they love you a lot, sometimes family members have the toughest time accepting the chronic illness of a loved one. Working with each individual to make the news more palatable helps, as does understanding the root cause for their hesitation or other negative reaction.

Parents' perspectives

There is no clear-cut genetic link that indicates that any one family member will definitely develop thyroid disease. But because it can run in families, that is, because blood relatives can share certain genetic components and sometimes develop thyroid disease, there can be a tendency to look upon genetics as the cause for the disease. Your parents might express feelings of guilt, denial, and even anger when you tell them about your diagnosis, especially if they feel that they were in some way responsible for your illness.

Denial can also be a component of how your parents react to your diagnosis. This is because they don't want you to be ill at all, and certainly not with a chronic illness. So they might ask you if your doctor could have "made a mistake." They might demonstrate their disbelief by expressing their dislike or wariness of the medical profession, saying, "What do doctors know, anyway?" They might try to persuade you to seek a second, third, even fourth opinion in their hopes that the doctors and lab tests are wrong.

Sometimes, parents turn on each other and accuse one another of "giving you" hypothyroidism, especially if a relative also has thyroid disease. This can cause tension at a time when you most need understanding and calm, so you're going to have to dig deep into your own internal resources for steadiness and understanding.

Conversely, parents might become too smothering, too horrified by your diagnosis. They might try to take over your healthcare, insisting that they know better than your physician does. Their overattention could cause you to pull away from them and move farther from the very support you need.

Before you tell your parents about your diagnosis, get a clear picture of your health condition and prognosis. Relate what you know as calmly as possible, and gently suggest that they learn about your condition, too, so that they can be supportive of you as you proceed with treatment. Reassure your parents that your illness is not terminal, that there is treatment for hypothyroidism. Be sensitive to their feelings of guilt, anguish, or confusion over your illness and help them accept it in their own time.

There's a fine line between explaining that hypothyroidism causes many of your symptoms and using your illness as an excuse not to address your problems. Instead of being accusatory or victimized, be positive about treating your thyroid imbalances in order to get back on track and avoid blaming anyone or anything for how you feel right now. Show your parents that you are a capable, strong adult and meet them on these terms. Over time, their misgivings will probably dissipate.

Sibling rivalry?

How your brothers and sisters relate to the news of your diagnosis depends greatly on what your overall relationship is with them. If your brother or sister has been jealous of you in the past, for example, the extra attention you receive as a result of your illness might cause him or her to resent you and act out this reaction in negative ways. This person, too, might deny that you have any illness at all and not offer support, emotional or otherwise, as you work through your symptoms and treatment.

Likewise, you might feel jealous that a brother or sister is healthy, whereas you have a chronic illness. You could ask, "Why me and not them?" and convey this resentment loudly enough so that they pick up on it and feel threatened by your frustration and anger. This could cloud your relationship and make it difficult, if not impossible, to nurture important familial bonds.

Sometimes, siblings might not want to acknowledge your disease for fear they themselves might contract it. They might even begin to neglect their own health, refusing to go to the doctor, for example, because they are so afraid.

In all of the above cases, try to be very understanding and careful to not give in to flaring emotions or one-upmanship. Explain your illness as calmly as you can. Encourage your siblings to take care of their own health, too, and help them understand the genetic component to hypothyroidism so that they will recognize symptoms if they occur but not be paranoid that they will definitely get sick themselves.

"For better, for worse . . ."

When one spouse is diagnosed with a chronic illness, the delicate balance of a marriage can become very lopsided. Suddenly, your chores might become your spouse's chores, expenses related to your illness might impact the whole family budget, and your ability to give 100 percent to your children, work, and intimacy with your partner might be completely undermined.

Your spouse might have a very difficult time accepting your illness because, up to this point, you weren't definitively diagnosed. Moreover, so many of the symptoms of hypothyroidism seem so "general" that they might not appear to be all that serious. For example, if you tell your husband you are constantly tired, he might reply that he is, too, instead of wondering if there is something medically wrong with you or offering the sympathy or consideration you desire.

Much like being rudely awakened, now that you know what you have and are seeking medical treatment for your condition, your spouse must come to terms with knowing that marriage is not always only "for better," but is also sometimes "for worse." He or she will have to make certain adjustments, including financial and personal, to accommodate the requirements of your symptoms and treatment. This could cause a rift between you, as you pay closer attention to your health and he pays closer attention to the problems it creates for the household. It also might bring you closer as you work together to make life meaningful and whole.

There is some validity to the notion that chronic illness is a major factor in couples getting divorced. But usually it is one component among several that drives the final wedge between a husband and a wife. It is, however, reasonable to assume that a marriage that is not strong to begin with will be sorely tested when one spouse becomes chronically ill.

Sometimes, divorce cannot be avoided. However before you take this sad step, take good stock of your marriage, the pros and cons, and what you can do to make it stronger. Communicate closely with your spouse about how you feel, and invite him or her to come with you to doctor's appointments so that he or she can feel part of your care. Work together to find ways to compensate for the limitations and problems illness brings into a home and intimate life, and try to keep a positive attitude toward it all, even amid pain and disappointment.

Yes, chronic illness can be a catalyst for a marriage to fall apart. But it can also be the thing that makes it stronger, more wonderful, and even more loving than it was before. Keep that in mind as you work through the rough times with your spouse. You will undoubtedly be glad you did.

Children

How much and when you tell your children that you are hypothyroid depends on their maturity and your attitude toward your diagnosis. Very young children might not understand the concept of illness, or they might jump to the conclusion that because you are ill you're going to die. They might become anxious and act out their fear in troubling ways, especially if you are nervous about your diagnosis and convey that, even unconsciously, when you tell them about it.

On the other hand, older children can better understand what you are going through and even help you cope with your condition. They have probably been exposed to the basics of science in school, so they can probably grasp the essentials of what hypothyroidism is, and they are usually more developed emotionally, too. The day-to-day management of your condition can be a tremendous learning tool for them. Relying on them to run errands for you or take care of the housework when you are too tired is an excellent way to teach compassion and care for someone else.

Be sensitive to how others, especially other children, might react to your children in light of your illness. That is, sometimes less sensitive people might single out your children because their parent is "different" or "sick all the time." Explaining to your children that some people don't understand can be difficult, but it can also help them gain a perspective on the world that can hold them in good stead as they become more experienced with coping with prejudice and bigotry.

Don't forget about you

Even if you have very young children and do not think it is appropriate to tell them you are hypothyroid, you should still take good care of your health. It does you and your family no good to pretend you are well when you aren't, or to ignore the needs of your body. Stick to your medication schedule and diet and exercise program, and keep current with your doctor's visits and lab tests. Being a parent is hard work, as you well know. You must be as strong as possible to be present for and to take care of your children.

Friends

When you suffer from the symptoms of hypothyroidism and are ultimately diagnosed with the chronic illness, you will truly get to know who your real friends are. Your illness can make you tired, so you might have to cancel plans to get together at the last minute. Hypothyroidism can also affect your appearance, so you might not look as attractive as you have in the past. Your depression or other emotional symptoms, especially mood swings, can be tough to deal with, and so unpredictable that you might not be very good company all the time.

Unlike family members, who are tied to you by blood or marriage, friends can come and go. Some will step right up and offer their support and help, making extra calls or asking to do things for you when you are especially low. Others, however, were not very firm friends to begin with. They will become impatient if you cancel plans too many times, and they might be very uneasy around you if you suffer from rashes, weight gain, and hair loss.

Friends who encourage you to do things that are not healthful are not friends at all. Anyone who wants you to "drown your sorrows" in excessive alcohol or illegal drug consumption isn't doing you any favors. Even on a more benign level, someone who is constantly trying to get you to try fad diets or other treatments can also be troublesome. You might have to withdraw from him or her, too, if you cannot reach an understanding that the course of treatment that you and your doctor have decided upon is best for you.

True friends are marvelous gifts. Be sure to treasure them, and be their friend as much as you want them to be your friends. If you have decreased energy and your emotions are fragile, surround yourself with friends who are positive, nurturing influences. Think of them, too, as "the best medicine."

Coworkers

If you have missed a lot of work because of your illness, or if your performance on the job has suffered because you have been depressed, lethargic, or moody, your coworkers might have built up a lot of resentment toward you. Looking at it from their point of view, because you have been functioning at less than 100 percent, they might have had to take on extra work and have not necessarily been paid more for doing it. In your pain and moodiness, you might have said something or behaved in a way to offend them, and your frustration might have caused further rifts between you.

In many workplaces, being part of a team is important. If you have a chronic illness and need special accommodation, such as time off to go to doctor's appointments or other physical consideration, you might be viewed by your coworkers in a negative light.

The first step toward trying to bring balance back into your work life is to be realistic and honest about what you have done or failed to do to be a good employee and part of your coworkers' team. Remember that they don't know what was going on inside your body, mind, and heart while you were suffering from the brunt of your symptoms; they only know what you did or said. Honesty is essential to successfully coping with your illness, and you must first be honest with yourself.

Next, you must speak with your supervisor about your desire to do your work and what, if any, accommodation you need to be able to perform it. Although you might not think of hypothyroidism as a disability (and, in fact, most people with the condition are never disabled from it), under the Americans with Disabilities Act (ADA), which covers workers for many of this country's employers, you are entitled to reasonable accommodation for your illness. (There are more details about the ADA in Week 4.)

Although there is certainly no stigma attached to being hypothyroid, don't feel you have to share the news of your diagnosis with everyone at work. Your supervisor is really the only person who needs to know your precise physical condition. Your health is your private, personal business. Still, if you decide to tell someone else, realize that even if you tell him or her in confidence, word has a way of "traveling" through the office, sometimes with undesirable consequences.

Remember the childhood game of "telephone"? Someone would whisper something to someone, who would whisper it to someone else, and so on down the line until the initial message was totally garbled. The same thing often happens in offices where the "grapevine" thrives. If you trust someone with the news of your diagnosis, your hypothyroidism might morph to something else as word of it moves from worker to worker. Decide carefully ahead of time if you really want and need other people you work with to know you are hypothyroid. Then, act and react appropriately.

If you experience personal conflicts on the job, seek help immediately to resolve them. Don't let bad feelings fester, and don't be a victim to someone else's ill will. Many times, personality conflicts are born out of misunderstanding, and a skilled mediator can help bring calm back into a charged work environment.

Above all, if you want to maintain a positive, working relationship with your employer and coworkers, try to be enthusiastic about working and try not to bring hypothyroidism into every aspect of your work. When you're at work, give 100 percent of your attention and effort. If you need time off or other accommodation, seek it with a sense of professionalism and cooperation.

Total strangers

This might seem like an odd heading to include in a section on telling people you know about your hypothyroidism. But, I kid you not, over the next few days, weeks, months, and years, at some point you will have conversations with total strangers about your condition. It's a little like walking around pregnant or getting your wisdom teeth out; everyone has a comment or story or knows someone who knows someone who knows someone who is hypothyroid.

These conversations might take place in the checkout line at the supermarket or in the waiting room at the doctor's office. Someone might ask you about your "weight problem" in an accusatory fashion, and you might be prompted to explain your struggle to cope with thyroid hormone imbalance. Someone else might ask you about the Synthroid you are picking up at the pharmacy.

News about hypothyroidism is in the press from time to time, and you will undoubtedly hear random comments about it and feel that you need to participate in the conversation. Someone might even strike up a conversation with you if they see you reading this book!

Decide how much you want to share about hypothyroidism early on. Don't feel as though you are a "poster child" for the illness, but if you are moved to explain something about it, feel free to do so. You probably aren't a medical expert, so you should avoid giving advice. But the more people understand about your condition, the more likely they will be to be supportive of others with it and the more likely they will be to support funding for research. Raising awareness of hypothyroidism can also help the estimated millions of people who go around with the condition without getting a diagnosis.[1] Remember when you were in that position? How wonderful it would be to help others on the road to better health!

IN A SENTENCE:

> *Whom you tell about your hypothyroidism is your decision, and how you tell others can enhance your support system tremendously.*

learning

The Meds

WHEN YOU are diagnosed with hypothyroidism, your doctor will probably suggest that you start your treatment with one of the types of pills that contain replacement thyroid hormone. These prescription medicines are divided into two principal categories: **natural** and **synthetic**. They are manufactured by several different pharmaceutical companies and vary in dosage, as well as in "look"—some are butterfly shaped, others are round, and each dosage usually has its own distinctive color.

Natural thyroid supplements

The earliest treatment for underactive thyroid was a serum containing sheep's thyroid. When this was administered, patients who had once exhibited the symptoms of hypothyroidism seemed to recover.[2] In the years that followed the first treatments for hypothyroidism, scientists sought to develop better and even more effective ways of delivering thyroid supplement to those people who needed it.

Today, there are several prescription preparations of natural thyroid supplements. All are in pill form and are formulated using desiccated pig's thyroid combined with other ingredients and binders (substances that hold all the ingredients of a pill together). Some examples of natural thyroid supplement include Nature-Thyroid and Westhroid, both manufactured by Western Research Laboratories, and Armour Thyroid, manufactured by Forest Pharmaceuticals, Inc. Although they are called "natural," they do come from animal thyroid glands, not human glands.

At present, there is no way to separate T_3 and T_4 from each other in the desiccated pig's thyroid, so natural thyroid hormone pills contain both. Because most patients do not need supplemental T_3 in addition to T_4, using natural thyroid hormone pills can cause some patients to have too much T_3 (active thyroid hormone) in their bodies, especially when the tablet they take is not standardized for T_3 content. They might run the risk of developing symptoms of hyperthyroidism, including tremors, heart palpitations, arrhythmias, and, over time, bone loss. Also, there are other components in natural thyroid hormone pills that cannot be separated out from the thyroid hormone itself, such as other organic substances present in the animal tissue.

If you decide to use one of the prescription natural thyroid supplements, you and your doctor should discuss the possibility of side effects, your ability to absorb the necessary amount of hormone, and monitor your T_4, T_3 *and* free T_3 levels to make sure you are keeping everything in balance. Also, if you are a vegan or vegetarian or have religious convictions that preclude you from eating pork, be aware that natural thyroid supplements do contain desiccated pig's thyroid, a direct animal product.

Synthetic thyroid hormone

In gemology, the term "synthetic" is used to describe a substance that is identical to the natural material, but is lab-created. So, a synthetic diamond has all of the chemical properties and crystal structure of a natural diamond, with the exception that, instead of originating and ultimately being mined from the ground or body of water, it was grown in a laboratory.

In the same way, medications that are not derived from animal or plant substances are considered synthetic, meaning they have the same properties as the natural substances, but are lab-produced. The synthetic thyroid hormone used to treat hypothyroidism is chemically the same as the hormone produced by your body and acts just as your own hormone does. Also, it does not have the other organic components of the natural thyroid hormone supplement, and so is more pure.

There are several brands of synthetic hormone. Among them are Synthroid (Abbott Laboratories), Levothyroid and Thyrolar Thyroid (Forest Pharmaceuticals, Inc.), Unithroid (Watson Pharma), and Levoxyl and Cytomel (King Pharmaceuticals). There is no generic form for Synthroid, however there is a generic form of Unithroid.

Each synthetic thyroid hormone pill contains one or both of the hormones specific to thyroid function, as well as other inactive ingredients and binders. Cytomel, for example, contains T_3. Thyrolar Thyroid contains both T_3 and T_4. Synthroid contains T_4.

Which medication you take depends on your individual situation, what your doctor recommends, and what hormones you need most. If you need to supplement both your T_4 and T_3, for example, you could use a product that has both in one tablet or take two different products, each with one of the hormones you need. If you don't need to supplement both T_4 and T_3, all you might need is medication that contains T_4.

The T_3/T_4 controversy

"The pendulum of treating hypothyroidism swings from only using T_4 to using T_4 and T_3 and back again," says Dr. Basil Rapoport, M.B., a research thyroidologist. "There is still debate over which is more effective, or which benefits the patient most. I'm sure the pendulum will swing several times before we have an answer. Above all, we must keep in mind that the first rule of medicine is to do no harm."

This distillation of years of opinions, professional and otherwise, to the various protocols used to treat hypothyroid patients is very useful to understand the continuity of medicine's approach to thyroid hormone supplements. Just as economic trends are cyclic, and some might say that social trends are cyclic (look at clothing fashions today and compare them to the 1970s!), trends in medicine can be cyclic, too.

The first natural thyroid supplements, from sheep's thyroid, contained both T_4 and T_3. Nowadays, the natural supplements from pig's thyroid also contain those two hormones. Some synthetic thyroid supplements contain only one of the hormones, and others contain both. Trends to use one or the other have ebbed and flowed over the years, and what is being considered now is no exception.

The literature on treating hypothyroidism is mixed as to which way is the best to go. Some physicians favor adding T_3 to the T_4 therapy, especially if the patient has been on T_4 but still complains of symptoms. Other physicians go strictly by TSH levels; as long as this component of measuring thyroid function is normal, there is no need to add more active hormone (T_3) or, for that matter, any T_4, either. Popular hypothyroid writings and experiences are mixed, too. I know some patients who are on "just" T_4 and others on that and T_3 as well. I myself have tried both therapies and because my thyroid is still in the process of "burning itself out," I can't say that I'm on my "ultimate" thyroid drug regimen, yet.

There are, of course, health considerations beyond hormone levels, which need to be considered when you are trying to work with your doctor to reach the optimum medication levels and types. Taking too much thyroid hormone could predispose you to complications such as **osteoporosis,** loss of bone mass, and heart **arrhythmias,** or irregular heartbeats.

As you research this area of thyroidology and read the pros and cons, as well as the personal anecdotes, keep in mind that your doctor is the one on whom you should be most reliant for advice and treatment. Our bodies are unique, and our physical makeups are individual, too. Although there is much popular literature about the benefits of T_3 therapy, a whole book of personal testimonies might not have anything to do with your particular situation—only your doctor will know for sure. As long as you have a physician who is willing to listen to you and monitor you correctly and carefully, you should rely upon him or her for your personal answer to the "T_4 or T_4/T_3?" question.

Herbal supplements

Apart from the prescription natural thyroid hormones mentioned here, there are no other herbal or plant derivatives that act in the same way and supplement thyroid hormone in people. That is not to say that someday there might be an animal-free, natural alternative to current medicines. But if anyone claims to have the plant-based solution to your thyroid problems, be very wary and discuss it thoroughly with your doctor before adding it to your thyroid treatment regimen. The same caution should be exercised with over-the-counter thyroid medications carried by health food stores.

Many of these contain kelp, which could damage your thyroid gland even more.

Depending on your overall health considerations, you might want to take other supplements. But before you take over-the-counter vitamins and herbs, check with your doctor and perhaps have a CBC panel done that tests the various vitamins and blood counts in your blood. This will indicate if you are deficient in any particular vitamin, and then you can be more specific as to which supplements you need to take.

Thyroid hormone and weight loss

Weight considerations are discussed in detail on Day 7, but for now, it is very important to know that reputable physicians agree that thyroid hormone should never be used to treat obesity. There are some diet programs that give out thyroid hormone, especially in high doses, to help their clients lose weight. This is a terrible idea, because giving thyroid hormone to people who do not need it for thyroid purposes runs the risk of dangerous side effects and significant damage to the thyroid gland itself. You should only take thyroid hormone because you need it to regulate your doctor-diagnosed hypothyroid condition.

Consistency is key

Usually, your doctor will recommend that you try to remain on the same brand of medication that you started on in order to get a correct read on how well the dosage and type of medication is working for you. This is especially true if you are taking generic levothyroxine, because different manufacturers of generic thyroid hormone might use different binders and substances to make their products.

Of course, if you have any adverse reactions to your pills, you should notify your doctor immediately. Sometimes, sensitivity to one medication might not be due to the active ingredients but rather to the binder used to keep the ingredients of a pill together. But whatever the reason, you need to work with your doctor to get the right treatment.

Staying with the same pharmacist for all your prescriptions and refills is an excellent idea. Many pharmacies have computers that will flag drug interactions based upon what you are being given, and they can also provide you with an end-of-the-year accounting of all your prescription expenses. Having one central pharmacist is good, too, because he or she will get to know you and can give you extra attention when you need it. And the convenience factor is very important—you don't want to expend your precious energy running from pharmacist to pharmacist!

Another area that you should try to keep consistent is what time of day you take your medication. This helps your body adjust to the supplemental hormone, and it also helps you get into the habit of taking your medication. Many of us are not used to taking pills on a daily, long-term basis. If you schedule taking your medication just as you would your daily workout, for example, you will be less likely to skip a dose. Also, keeping your medication in the same place at home will save you from having to expend energy searching for your pills.

If you miss a dose

Until recently, physicians, pharmacists, and pharmaceutical companies advised patients against doubling up on days after missing a dose of supplemental thyroid hormone. However, at a recent meeting of the American Thyroid Association, Gilbert H. Daniels, M.D., gave a presentation on treating hypothyroidism where he said, "When a dosage of levothyroxine is missed, two pills may (should) be taken the next day. If two pills are missed, three may be taken on the third day."[3] This information is very useful, especially for a patient who has trouble complying with an everyday regimen (which is the ideal). But before you double up on your thyroid medication, you should speak with your doctor about whether it is all right for you to do so.

Quality control

Recently, there has been a lot of press about thyroid hormone manufacturers and the Food and Drug Administration's (FDA) approval of their products used to treat hypothyroidism. Some people might have concerns that their medications are not stable, or do not give accurate dosages. This is what's been going on.

Hypothyroidism was first recognized in the 1800s, and Hashimoto's thyroiditis was first identified as an autoimmune disease in 1912. Some of the first thyroid supplement was serum made of sheep's thyroid, and this was used until pill form of thyroid hormone was developed.

Many of the current synthetic thyroid hormone medications in pill form that are used to treat hypothyroidism were used as long ago as the 1950s. Because they have been used for so long, they were "grandfathered" into the FDA's approved list of drugs and did not have to go through the stringent approval process that most other drugs must undergo.

In 1997, however, the FDA decided that there was some concern about the manufacturing process of thyroid hormone supplements, as well as the consistency of their dosages and the stability of their shelf life and potential side effects. The FDA told all manufacturers of supplemental thyroid hormone medications that they had to go through an approval process to continue marketing their products to patients. This included review of the manufacturing process to ensure that the pills produced were stable and contained the amount of hormone that they were supposed to have.

As of October 2002, thyroid hormone manufacturers are going or have gone through the approval process. Many of these, including the manufacturers of Levo-T, Levoxyl, Novothyrox, Synthroid, and Unithroid, have made the FDA's recommended adjustments so that their products can be prescribed for and provided to hypothyroid patients. Updates to the approved list are available on the FDA's Web site (*www.fda.gov*) and through the American Thyroid Association and the Thyroid Foundation of America. Your doctor, too, should be vigilant about the latest in the FDA's approvals and prescribe dosages and brands of medications for you accordingly.

Over-the-counter remedies, including health food store herbs, do not have to go through the FDA's approval process. As a result, the efficacy of the preparations, as well as their contents and potency, can vary from brand to brand and batch to batch. If you decide to take any herbal or other over-the-counter preparations, be sure that you check first with your doctor to ensure that you are not doing yourself any harm or causing any drug interactions before going ahead. If you purchase preparations abroad, be aware that the ingredients might not be comparable to those used in medications in the U.S. and could be harmful to you.

Your role in medication therapy

Thyroid medications are prescribed by your doctor, and the prescriptions are filled by a registered pharmacist. But there are things that you can do, too, so that you get the most from your medication therapy.

Whenever you get a new prescription, ask your doctor and pharmacist if there are any potential side effects related to the medication they are giving you. If you notice any of these, notify your doctor immediately.

Ask your doctor and pharmacist if there are any food or drug interactions you need to be aware of and schedule taking your medication accordingly. For example, thyroid hormone should not be taken at the same time as calcium supplements because calcium might deter the absorption of supplemental thyroid hormone. The action of certain other medications, such as anti-psychotic drugs, can be affected if taken at the same time as thyroid medication. Antacids might prevent proper absorption of thyroid hormone, and so should not be taken at the same time as thyroid medication.

It is always a good idea to tell your doctor and pharmacist about all the medications you are taking so that he or she can give you informed answers to your questions about interactions and make any necessary modifications to your medication regimen. Be wary of anyone who encourages you to take a "natural" herb or supplement without getting your doctor's approval; even natural substances have chemical components that can interact with what you are being prescribed.

In general, store your medication in a place that is dry and free from severe temperature fluctuations. For example, keeping it above your stove is probably not a good idea, nor is keeping it in the medicine cabinet in your bathroom. But keeping it in a cupboard in your kitchen that is farther away from heat sources, or in a drawer in your bedroom dresser, might be all right. Ask your pharmacist if you should do anything special to store your medication. Some (such as Thyrolar Thyroid) are highly sensitive to temperature fluctuations and might require refrigeration.

Try to stay ahead of your refills, making sure that you would still have enough medication if you couldn't go to the pharmacy for a few days. Thankfully, emergencies don't occur every day. But if there were an earthquake, or snowstorm, or if you fell ill and could not get your medication, you could experience adverse affects. An extra precaution is to locate a pharmacy that delivers. The added cost you incur for this service is worth the peace of mind and continuity of healthcare that keeping your supply of medication coming will give you.

How long does it take for the meds to kick in?

Some hypothyroid patients say that it only took a week or two for them to feel better after starting on thyroid medication. Others say it took longer. Sometimes, patients feel better, but not completely so, and have to work with their doctors to adjust the dosages or combination of hormones they take. With a disease such as Hashimoto's thyroiditis, where the gland "burns it out," it can take months or years to ultimately get to the right dosage of thyroid hormone. This might be due to the fact that the thyroid gland fails slowly over time. Other patients might have overlapping illnesses that make it difficult to determine exactly what symptoms are due to hypothyroidism and what are due to their other conditions.

There can be a kind of "roller coaster" effect, too, that includes your thrill at finally being treated for your illness and the effects of thyroid hormones on your system, as well as your thyroid gland's function. You might, for example, feel very happy and well in the first days following your diagnosis, when you start your medication and know that you're taking a positive step toward wellness. But after a couple of weeks, you might start to feel low as the realization hits you that you have an ongoing medical condition, and one that causes other symptoms besides just feeling lethargic. Your mood might swing back and forth, making you wonder if, having taken control, you really are in control.

Patience, patience

Getting used to the ups and downs of hypothyroidism takes fortitude, courage, and a lot of patience. I'm not the most patient person in the world (ask my friends!), so I developed some techniques to help me cope.

One of the most important things I do is pray and meditate. This helps my mind and body to relax and fills my spirit with calm and comfort. In meditation, for example, I try to focus on something with a very slow pace. One of my favorite things is to imagine myself sitting beside the ocean on a starlit Hawaiian night. I'm not running, not working, not even thinking of my hypothyroidism. I'm just sitting—and helping myself disconnect from the more frantic world around me and my inner feelings of impatience.

I also tend to do some things on certain days. For example, on Wednesdays and Saturdays, I try to tend to my houseplants. Knowing that I'll be doing this helps me punctuate the days of a week and gives me small "goals" to accomplish while I am waiting for the larger picture to unfold.

Talking about being impatient helps me to articulate my desire to have time move more quickly or for a particular medication or treatment to work faster. I try not to be a burden to my family and friends, but it does help! Also, having enjoyable things to do and beloved people to spend time with helps make the moment as important as the future. It's hard to realize this, I know, because we live in such a goal-oriented society. But there is much truth in the statement, "Any day I can get out of bed, breathe, and look outside is a very good day."

IN A SENTENCE:

> *Hypothyroidism can be treated with a variety of prescription thyroid hormone supplements, and you need to use patience, consistency, and doctor-patient communication and cooperation to make your hypothyroid treatment work.*

Lingering Emotional Effects of Hypothyroidism

BY NOW, your initial feelings of relief and determination to take charge of your health might have faded somewhat as you realize the extent to which hypothyroidism has and will continue to affect your life. Although you have begun taking medication, you have yet to experience relief. You probably notice that your weight gain did not disappear the day you started taking your medication, and your hair did not grow back overnight. Your nails and skin are still problematic, and the cloud of depression that was so oppressive before your diagnosis is still there, pulling your mood and determination down at a time when you need it most. You have begun to tell your family and friends about your condition and their reactions have comforted, surprised, and maybe even dismayed you. You might even fear that some of your relationships will never be as good as they were before you became ill. And as for your fatigue, well, it's as present and oppressing as ever.

Letting go to move forward

In many ways, accepting that you have a chronic illness means having to let go of your old way of life and take up a completely different one. In your old life, you didn't have to take medication, and you had ample energy, vitality, fitness, and hope for the future. You didn't need to budget for doctor's visits, medication, and other health-related items. You didn't have to keep to a medication schedule. Being sick meant having a cold, the flu, or breaking your leg . . . and recovering from it.

But now you are hypothyroid, and you know that in all likelihood your health will have to be monitored and you will need to take medication for the rest of your life. You *do* have to budget for all this, fit it into your schedule, and be more careful of what you eat and how you take care of yourself. You'll have to work much harder at feeling well, at keeping your body and mind fit. And all of this will separate you a little from your more able-bodied friends and family members. Not everyone will understand what you are going through, and not everyone will want to listen to you as you explain it. You might lose friends, relationships, and your sense of wellness.

But for all the negative things happening in your life, if you are reading this book, you already know that you have a tremendous desire to learn about your health condition and do something about it. Even before you started reading this book, by pursuing your diagnosis, you were taking care of yourself in a way that few people have had to do. You have demonstrated that you are ready to face the future with hypothyroidism.

To do this, you will, in many significant ways, have to say good-bye to the past and embrace the future. All the emotions associated with this transition will take time to work through. As with mourning the loss of a loved one, you will find that you don't go through these emotions in any particular order, and might swing back and forth among them for a while. The more you understand about how you feel, the better you will be able to cope.

Sorrow

We live in a time when we're always told to "look on the bright side." As you share the news of your diagnosis, some people will undoubtedly tell you to "cheer up," pointing out that your health problem isn't as serious as other people's troubles. After all, hypothyroidism isn't terminal.

But you well know that having a chronic illness means letting go of full health and is in a sense like saying good-bye to a beloved friend. Yes, hypothyroidism is not as horrific as some other illnesses. It is not fatal, and should not take over your whole existence. But it *is* a life-altering, ongoing illness that will bring many changes to your life.

When you think of your life this way, you might be struck by many feelings, especially sadness and sorrow. Much like when you are mourning the loss of a loved one, sorrow doesn't well up all at once and then dissipate forever. It takes time for sadness to abate. Indeed, working through your sadness is a process, and you need to be patient and loving with yourself while you do it.

The process of coping with sorrow begins with recognizing that you feel sadness and that it is connected with your illness. It isn't the song on the radio that's making you sad, and it isn't something your friend said to you. No, you are sorrowful because you have an illness that will not go away. There's nothing wrong with feeling like this; you're in good company with most of us who were diagnosed with hypothyroidism. You're human. You are sad. That's okay.

After facing the root of your sadness, you will probably want to express your sorrow, to "let it out" so that you can move through it. Writing about your emotions in your health journal is one way to express your sadness. So is talking with trusted loved ones. You might feel like punching a pillow or curling up in the fetal position on your bed. You might cry. You might cry a lot. That is okay, too. In fact, I think that the benefit of crying is overlooked many times when we are trying to work through our negative feelings in today's world. Crying is a very real, outward manifestation of the heart's sadness, and it can help cleanse ourselves emotionally so that we can face the future squarely.

Whether you are a man or a woman who has been diagnosed with hypothyroidism, it is all right to say you are sad. It is all right to express your sorrow. Eventually, your tears will subside, just as your sorrow does. You will feel stronger about your ability to meet the challenges of hypothyroidism. You will understand your body better, and your medication will be more effective. There *is* a better day ahead. But right now, it's perfectly all right to cry.

Frustration and impatience

Much of the frustration you feel when you begin treatment for hypothyroidism has to do with the delay between when you start to take the pills and when you sense an improvement. Some of this is because of the way the medication works. You probably won't suddenly wake up one day and all your symptoms will be gone. Rather, you have to wait days, weeks, or perhaps even months before you start to feel better. Adjusting your dosage of thyroid medication can be an ongoing process, sometimes taking years as your thyroid gland burns itself out. And then there are the lingering physical effects that can sometimes be even harder to cope with and take longer to go away.

Frustration takes many outward guises and can exacerbate symptoms that you already have. Tension might build up in your muscles and cause you pain. If you already have fibromyalgia or arthritis, this can make you feel worse than you usually do, inhibit your ability to exercise, and interfere with your sleep. You could also become frustrated with friends or family members, especially if they seem to be pushing you to say you are feeling better or that your hypothyroidism "is over." Other people might relate stories to you about others who had seemingly immediate success with their treatment, and this could make you wonder if your doctor is doing the right thing, or if you are doing something wrong.

Examine your activities and thoughts closely if you suspect there might be some truth to wondering if you are doing something wrong in your quest to make yourself feel better. Some people rely on "comfort" activities if they are frustrated with the speed or quality of how their thyroid treatment is working, and these actions might do more harm than good. Binge eating fatty or high-carbohydrate foods is one of these activities, and it can be harmful because it can lead to more weight gain, high cholesterol, and other health problems. Giving yourself a sugar high because you are tired will stress your body and can lead to more fatigue and weight gain.

Just as with binge eating, impulse shopping, consuming inappropriate amounts of alcohol, taking illegal drugs, or risking your physical and emotional safety can also be manifestations of your frustration and anger. Be aware of this and gauge your reactions to your illness carefully so that you don't fall into one or another of these harmful activities. Be careful, too, that you do not push yourself to engage in sex at a time when you do not feel "in the mood." Low thyroid function can have a negative effect on libido, and this can cause friction between partners. However, it is never a good idea to engage in sexual activity if you do not want to. Open communication and understanding are key for getting over this sensitive time between partners. Finding alternatives to promote intimacy and express the love between you and your partner is also important, and can help you both discover new and satisfying ways of relating to one another.

Practicing meditation and/or prayer and keeping a positive attitude can also be extremely important in ridding yourself of uncomfortable frustration. Turning your negative emotions into positive thoughts, dreams, and activities will go a long way toward making you more comfortable with how your individual thyroid treatment is progressing. Setting achievable goals at work and at home can help you maintain your sense of accomplishment as you physically struggle to get back to "the way you were" before you became ill.

Bargaining

One of the most potentially dangerous aspects of dealing with the loss of our health and the need to move into the future with a chronic illness is the bargaining many of us do with our doctors, ourselves, and even God. This way of setting unrealistic goals is natural to do; we want to feel that we are in control of our lives even if our health is out of our sphere of influence. But bargaining can backfire, increasing frustration, impatience, and lowering our self-worth.

You can identify bargaining by noticing if you use a sentence or sentences with the construction, "If" . . . "then."

"I'll take this pill for three months. But if I'm not feeling better, then I'll stop because it means I'm really not hypothyroid." This attitude reflects denial and leaves the door open for extreme disappointment at the end of the "bargained" time period.

"If I accept that I have hypothyroidism, then God will make my life easier, right?" This bargain sets up an unrealistic future; no life is without challenges, and God doesn't make life easier because someone has a chronic illness.

"It doesn't matter if I eat nutritiously because I'm only a little hypothyroid. If my condition gets worse, then I'll think about changing my diet." This attitude invites bad dietary habits, which can lead to weight gain, lower self-esteem, and a cycle of unhealthful living.

The temptation to bargain comes from an unwillingness to accept illness. We all have to watch out for the tendency to bargain away our responsibility toward our bodies and our health. Thyroid medication is serious business, as is making sure that our bodies are as healthy as they can be. Accepting your role in your healthcare is vitally important to being able to achieve a desirable, positive quality of life.

Being positive

"I'm a very positive person," says Rachel W., who is hypothyroid and has been treated for thyroid cancer. "I am always grateful. My attitude is that it could always be worse."

When you hear a hypothyroid patient say this, and you yourself are suffering greatly, you might be tempted to dismiss these words as "pie in the sky" or trite. However some people *are* positive by their very nature. No matter what challenges life throws at them, they see the sunny side, the glass half full. This doesn't mean that these people are ignoring their health problems or making light of the seriousness of their condition. We never know what's really going on inside someone; chances are they've gone through their share of fears, frustration, and confusion. But they make a choice, conscious or unconscious, to make the best of their troubles.

Listening to what Rachel W. and other hypothyroids say helps you to realize that there is another way to approach your condition besides dwelling on the negative. It takes practice, but it is possible to change your way of thinking about adversity. If you think before you speak (or complain) and are very vigilant about not allowing yourself to immediately latch on to what is most painful or terrible about your life, you can begin to take charge of your well-being in a positive way. And as you work through your emotions, in your own time and in your new, fresh way, you will move away from negative bargaining and begin to approach your healthcare from a position of strength and resilience. And you will find many "gifts" among the challenges.

IN A SENTENCE:

> *The emotional effects of your diagnosis are completely individual to you and might include frustration, impatience, sorrow, and bargaining; however, you can learn to cope with them and adopt a healthy positive attitude that will help you resolve them.*

learning

Everything's Affected

IN SUBSTANTIAL and subtle ways, your lowered metabolism has had an effect on almost every aspect of your life. Your emotions, physical stamina and energy, relationships with others, and your ability to give 100 percent to your job and household—all come into play when you are hypothyroid. Moreover, how you respond to your illness and seek help for your problems has great bearing on how well you will cope.

Recognizing how each aspect of your life has been affected and taking steps to correct any negative impact will help you mend fences and regain a sense of self-worth and accomplishment, which also have been impacted by your hypothyroidism. Today, we'll look at the various areas of your health, body, and life that could be affected by hypothyroidism. In the days and weeks that follow, we'll delve into specific ways to cope with each of them. Know that you might not experience all of these affects; I have included all of them so that each patient can recognize some of the things that might affect him or her.

Starting with metabolism

Your **metabolism** is a finely tuned system of chemical and physical processes within your body that regulates the rate at which your body grows, develops, and operates. Metabolism happens in two phases: the **anabolic** and the **catabolic** phase. Think of them as the "building up" and the "breaking down" of the nutrients and energy associated with keeping your body going. In the anabolic phase, the complex nutrients you take in are broken down into less complex substances and used to build up cells so that they can properly function and grow. In the catabolic phase, these substances are broken down once again by the cells, producing the energy (or "fuel") that keeps your body and its organs going. The pace at which this process moves is called your **metabolic rate**.

You can increase your metabolic rate by several means, including exercise or raising your body temperature. Your thyroid hormones play an integral part in regulating your metabolic rate, too. Any variation in thyroid hormone production, either up or down, will affect the whole chain of processes that fuel your body. If you are hyperthyroid, your metabolic rate will increase. If you are hypothyroid, your metabolic rate will fall.

A slower metabolic rate affects the pace at which your digestion works, your heart pumps blood, and your brain processes information. It also affects your sensitivity to cold; have you noticed that when you are hypothyroid, you often have difficulty getting warm? Many hypothyroid patients have body temperatures that are lower than the normal base of 98.6° F. This is because your metabolism has slowed down and less "heat" is being thrown off by your body, inside and out.

Weight and digestion

As you became increasingly hypothyroid, you might have gained weight and had more difficulty losing it. This is directly linked to your slower metabolism—you simply are not processing food as quickly as you should. In addition, you could get severely constipated and bloated, which will further give you the feeling that you are "blimping out." Still, even with the direct relationship between weight gain and thyroid imbalance, the issue is a complex one.

Many hypothyroid patients attribute all of their weight gain (even hundreds of extra pounds) to their thyroid problems. In practice, however, weight gain as a direct result of hypothyroidism is usually between five and ten pounds. Weight gain over this amount is generally not attributed solely to an underactive thyroid. Other factors that come into play include emotional responses to life in general and health in particular, lack of knowledge and practice of what constitutes a proper diet, overeating, and lack of appropriate exercise.

"Often, I ask a patient if anyone else in their family has thyroid problems and they'll say, 'my uncle so-and-so weighed three hundred pounds, so he must have had a thyroid problem,'" says Elliot Levy, M.D., a professor of medicine and thyroidologist. "But usually, that kind of weight gain is not because of a thyroid problem at all."

As you treat your hypothyroidism, your body will adjust to a more healthful metabolic rate, and you will be able to metabolize food properly once again. Some of the other circumstances that caused you to gain additional weight will need to be addressed as well so that you can achieve and maintain a healthful weight and body fat ratio. Your thyroid medication is not, in any way, intended to be used as a weight loss or weight maintenance drug.

Hair loss

Losing hair is a natural part of our lives. According to the American Academy of Dermatology, typical daily hair loss for each person is between 60 and 100 hairs. This is because of the growth cycle of our **hair follicles**, the tiny organs in our scalp and elsewhere on our body from which single hairs grow. It takes about four to five years for a hair to grow to its full length (hair grows about half an inch each month). After that time, the hair "rests" for between two and three months. Then the body sheds it and a new hair begins to grow from the same follicle. Most of the hair on your scalp is in its growing cycle; approximately 10 percent is "at rest."[1]

As you age, fewer follicles regenerate, causing your hair to thin. Sometimes, however, the normal growth cycle of your hair is disturbed, and you lose more hair than is normal. There are many reasons for this.

Alopecia is the medical term for hair loss. The most common type is **androgenic** alopecia, which is an inherited condition; male pattern baldness (and women pattern baldness) is androgenic alopeciae. Today, there is nothing much you can do to prevent androgenic alopecia; your propensity to lose your hair in this manner is programmed in your genes. Treating it is usually unhelpful, however you might find comfort in wigs, toupees, or possibly surgery.

Another cause of abnormal hair loss is an autoimmune disease, which has three subsets: **Alopecia areata, alopecia totalis, and alopecia universalis.**

In alopecia areata, hair loss is confined to one or more specific locations on the body (usually the head). Usually, the loss is in a round "clump" that pulls out of the head and leaves a smooth, round scalp surface. In alopecia totalis, all of the hair on the scalp falls out, leaving the person completely bald.

The most extreme form of autoimmune hair loss is alopecia universalis. This is a disease where a person loses all the hair on his or her body, except sometimes the pubic hair.

Alopeciae areata, totalis, and universalis are caused by antibodies that attack the hair follicles. Sometimes the hair doesn't grow for several years, and sometimes it never grows back. Various treatments are often offered to the patient suffering from one of these diseases. These include injections of cortisone and the use of topical creams, such as Rogaine or Propecia. Sometimes oral steroids are used in conjunction with one of these treatments, especially if the patient suffers from one or more internal autoimmune diseases.

Other causes of hair loss are:

- vitamin and nutrient deficiencies
- infection and disease
- stress and/or catastrophic life event (divorce, change of job, birth or death of a loved one, accident)
- medications (chemotherapy)
- surgery
- aftermath of pregnancy
- hormone imbalance (including hypothyroidism, which can affect hair growth and the ability of the follicles to produce hair and regenerate.)

Typically, hair loss from hypothyroidism manifests in finding more hairs on your comb or in your brush, or in the shower drain. Also, some patients lose both of their lateral eyebrows. This happened to me, and my endocrinologist wanted to get her camera and take a picture; in all her years of practice, she told me she'd only seen two patients who presented with this reportedly "classic" effect of hypothyroidism.

If you experience "clumplike" hair loss, you might have alopecia areata instead, or you might be genetically programmed to lose your hair as you age. It is best to report unusual hair loss to your doctor immediately so that you can investigate what the cause for it might be. Although it's sometimes convenient to "blame" everything on the thyroid gland, sometimes a patient can have multiple illnesses. You are much better off investigating each symptom, especially hair loss, to make sure you and your doctor are not overlooking anything.

Cholesterol

Hypothyroidism can affect the ability of your body to absorb what you eat healthfully, and you could develop high cholesterol levels, especially high "bad" cholesterol (LDL). This can cause arterial and heart complications, so you must be particularly careful about what you eat while you are waiting for your thyroid levels to come back into the normal range. Usually, with a good diet and regulated thyroid levels, your cholesterol levels will remain steady, too.

Skin

Your skin is the largest organ that you have. It protects your internal body from bacteria and other potentially fatal damage, helps your body regulate its temperature, and, with external secreting glands, helps to rid your body of moisture and impurities.

With all of the internal changes that go on in your body because of hypothyroidism, it is no wonder that your outer self, your skin, is affected, too. In fact, your skin relies on your thyroid gland to function properly, just as your other organs do. And when it is adversely affected, it can manifest everything from flaking to rashes and dryness to itching. These and other problems, from head to toe, can become one of the most uncomfortable and unsightly parts of your hypothyroidism. But they can also mimic other problems, besides hypothyroidism, including psoriasis, an infection or another illness, or allergy.

It is very important that you work with your doctor and, if possible, a **dermatologist** (a doctor who specializes in treatment of the skin, hair, and scalp) to determine the exact nature of your skin problems. The sooner you identify what is causing your discomfort, the sooner you'll be able to take steps to treat it.

Muscle strength

Muscles help the body and its organs to move. They propel us as we walk, lift, and stretch, and they play integral roles in making our heart muscle, lungs, and digestive systems move, too. Muscles are really collections, or bundles, of cells (also called "fibers"). They too rely on your thyroid gland to regulate the metabolism that, in turn, regulates their functioning. If your thyroid gland fails to produce enough hormone to charge your metabolism, then your muscles will not be able to move as strongly or as well as they should. This can lead directly to loss of muscle strength, as well as other problems, especially muscle cramps.

Another reason for loss of muscle strength is fatigue. If you are hypothyroid, you might be very tired. Fatigue, added to some of your other symptoms such as depression, might lead you to be more sedentary or to spend more time in bed. This means that you do not get as much exercise as you would if you were healthy and could contribute to loss of muscle strength and tone. Cramping, particularly in the calves and feet, common in hypothyroid patients, can also impede your ability to exercise fully.

Mind

Many hypothyroid patients complain of something they call "brain fog." It manifests itself in different ways, including difficulty concentrating, short attention span, memory lapses, and a general sense of being detached from the world around you. This is also due to a slower metabolism and lack of enough thyroid hormone to stimulate the blood vessels and cells that relate to brain function. Most times, after a patient is on an appropriate dosage of medication, his or her brain fog will clear up. It might recur if hypothyroid symptoms come back, but generally it is not permanent.

Mood

As many women who suffer from premenstrual syndrome (PMS) know, any surge or decrease in hormones can bring on a storm of various moods. In fact, many women report that they feel considerably worse during PMS when they are hypothyroid. Men, too, notice that they are more moody if they have a thyroid imbalance.

Moodiness due to thyroid imbalance must be separated from depression or other psychological problems in order to be addressed and, if necessary, treated. Keeping a health journal where you can track your mood swings and the reasons for them will help you and your doctor pinpoint exactly what is causing them. So, too, will listening to trusted loved ones when they bring up how "differently" you seem to be behaving. Sometimes others can notice things that escape us when we are ill or less than functional.

Fertility/libido

"I totally lost my sex drive from being hypothyroid," says Lidia Q. "My husband and I used to be like bunnies. Then, for about a year and a half, there was nothing going on."

Hypothyroidism has a direct effect on your libido and can also hinder your ability to conceive or carry a pregnancy to term. Some of the effect on the libido is due to psychological reasons: you feel unattractive because your appearance has changed so much, or you are afraid your partner will be repulsed if he or she gets close to you and sees the changes in your appearance. More influential, however, is the effect the decrease in thyroid hormone has on the responses and hormones that make up your sex drive. When your thyroid is underactive, your whole body slows down.

Fertility, too, can be affected by hypothyroidism. Your period might become very irregular, making it difficult to determine when you can conceive during your menstrual cycle. If you do conceive, your lack of appropriate thyroid hormone could affect the ability of your body to hold on to the fetus.

Any woman who believes she is or wants to become pregnant should have her thyroid gland checked. Discovering that you are hypothyroid can save a lot of money and heartache that might go toward multiple treatments to encourage fertility.

If your libido is low or nonexistent, a thyroid check should be done, too. In addition, other tests and examinations should be done to make sure that there are no other factors at play in either a case of infertility or low sex drive.

IN A SENTENCE:

> *Recognize the areas of your life that seem to be symptomatic of hypothyroidism, get a firm diagnosis of what is causing them, and make a game plan to do something about them.*

Identifying Cycles

EACH DAY, we participate in and are affected by cycles. Economic cycles. Social cycles. Eating cycles. Sleep cycles. Emotional cycles. There are many different varieties, beneficial and not-so-beneficial. They all ebb and flow in a certain pattern and are usually stimulated by a simple or complex association of cause and effect.

From a health perspective, on a good day when you feel strong, everything seems to go along well, as if the world is in sync with your body, mind, and spirit. But when you are not feeling well, even the slightest inconvenience can derail your day and lead you to get enmeshed in cycles that are not good for you. Bad habits, we might call them. Or worse, some kinds of addictions that are difficult to get free of, as much as we try. As a hypothyroid patient, for example, your condition might cause you to become depressed. This hormonal imbalance–induced depression can be made worse by your unhappiness at the physical changes you see in the mirror—the hair loss, the flaky skin—and by the emotional mood swings and loss of attraction to your husband or wife. The fatigue caused by your condition might exacerbate all of these things, and you might sink even lower. And when this happens, you might begin to do things that work against your good health.

When some people are depressed, they might binge on unhealthy foods, such as chocolate, cakes, or fatty, high-carbohydrate pastas with oil-laden sauces. These "comfort" foods taste good and in some cases hearken back to childhood, when the world seemed brighter. But as warmly nostalgic as they might make you feel, these kinds of foods cause you to run the risk of gaining weight, increasing your cholesterol levels, and possibly even raising your blood sugar to dangerous heights. As you feel worse from un-nutritious eating you could become more despondent and eat even more—falling deeper into an unhealthful cycle.

Another negative cycle might arise from the lack of self-esteem you might feel because of all the physical changes that take place with reduced thyroid hormone levels. With the hair loss, skin problems, and weight gain associated with hypothyroidism, your body image could suffer and you might feel completely unattractive to your spouse or partner. Also, hormonal imbalances could cause your libido to be greatly reduced or, in some cases, nonexistent. You might find yourself "acting out" your frustrations verbally or physically, saying and doing things that hurt your partner. He or she might lash back at you, and you might retaliate. All too quickly, you could fall into a cycle of hurtful emotions and damage the very person whom you love and upon whom you need to rely on more than ever. Or, you might go to the opposite extreme and try even harder to satisfy your partner, engaging in sexual or other activity that you truly have no desire to participate in. Lowering your ability to draw boundaries and taking part in physical activities that you have no desire to engage in can lead to a cycle of abuse that can further weigh you down.

Procrastination can lead to cycles that wreak havoc on your body and mind. If you are tired one day, you might put off exercising to the next. But on that day, you might be even less inclined to move around and put off exercising again. Too much procrastination can take you so far away from your exercise or other goals that they eventually seem unattainable. You might even stop thinking of exercise altogether, a result of an unhealthy cycle that is not desirable for anyone, let alone a hypothyroid patient.

The reverse of being idle is to approach your hypothyroidism in a frantic sort of way, forcing yourself to be hyperactive and then "crashing and burning" when you finish what you are doing and take the time to rest.

"Before I was diagnosed, it was almost a manic time," says Joe R., who is self-employed. "I would hold back the pain and fatigue and work real hard to get something done. Afterward, I would crash and burn. This cyclical thing of getting it together, working hard, and crashing and burning created a real negative feedback. I wondered, 'If this is what I have to do to do what I want to do and what I get in return is pain, is it worth it?'"

Identifying cycles

The first step toward being able to break a harmful cycle is to realize that you're in one. You need to be completely truthful with yourself. Realize, for example, that "just one more" piece of chocolate cake doesn't usually stop there, but rather leads to "just one more and more and more." On a calendar, keep track of the days when you don't exercise. This will help you see how much you are turning away from this healthful activity and how much saying, "I'm not going to do it today," can lead to weeks and months of detrimental inactivity.

When you have a chronic illness, you need to be extra sensitive to your body, your medical condition, and your emotional strength at all times. If you feel particularly unattractive and your loved one is in a "bad mood," try to disengage yourself from him or her for a little while instead of pushing yourself or your partner to give emotionally what they, or you, cannot give at the moment. Maintain communication through these episodes, being careful not to put the blame on yourself or your partner. Remember, no one is to blame for how you feel.

Just as important as recognizing what's going on inside of you is to acknowledge that you don't have control over how someone else feels, but you do have control over how you react to your symptoms and your and your loved one's emotions. Being accusatory of your loved one's seeming indifference to how you feel ("You just don't care," "You just don't understand") doesn't help turn around a volatile situation. But communicating gently ("I really need for you to understand what's going on with me") and meeting your partner halfway ("I know you want to do _____, but I honestly can't. Instead, let's do _____") will help open up solid channels of communication. And if, after you and your partner have tried to make your relationship better, it remains strained, don't hesitate to speak with your doctor about counselors or therapists he or she knows who work with couples coping with a chronic illness that's causing problems in their relationship.

Keep a health journal

I already mentioned one use for keeping a health journal, which is to keep track of your mood swings so that you can work with your doctor to identify possible causes for them. You can also use a health journal to identify when you seem to fall into bad habits or cycles—what triggers you to move into them and what helps you get out of them.

A health journal need not be elaborate or complicated. You can purchase a blank notebook or use sheets of paper and put them into a three-ring binder. Start with the current day and write down the "facts": what symptoms you have, what medication you are on, how you seem to be responding to the medication, your weight, your temperature (take it at the same time each day), and anything else pertaining to your condition. Next, write about your thoughts and feelings. Look upon this as a diary, as well as a health "log" and write down what makes you angry, sad, happy, and fulfilled, as well as what seems to affect your symptoms.

Along with your feelings and symptoms, include any outside factors that might influence them. Was it a sunny or rainy day? Did you receive a great piece of news? Did you have to wait in a long line at the supermarket and became anxious as a result? Keep a tally of all the foods you eat each day. Include snacks, "bites," and anytime you picked off "just a taste" of something. Make note of the beverages you drink (glasses of water, sips of vodka . . . don't leave anything out!) and include your feelings when you ate and drank. Were you depressed, frustrated, or hungry? Did your anger make you eat more quickly and thus take in more calories than you should have? Were you drinking wine alone, or in the company of loved ones. Did anyone remark that it seemed you had had too much to drink?

When you have written down everything for that day, look back and try to quantify your symptoms and feelings. Use a scale of 1 to 10, with "1" being lowest and "10" being highest or strongest. For example, was your muscle weakness really bad ("8" on a scale of 1 to 10) or moderate ("5" on a scale of 1 to 10)? Were you very angry with your friend because he said something hurtful ("7" on the scale) or were you livid ("9" on the scale)?

SAMPLE HEALTH JOURNAL

HEALTH FACTS

(Note the specifics of each item listed)

Day/Time:

Temperature: Weight:

Medications: Other healthcare facts:

FEELINGS AND SYMPTOMS

(After you have listed things in these columns, give them a numerical value, with "10" being the highest or best and "1" being the least or worst)

General Feeling (strong, weak, bloated, "foggy", etc.):

Specific Symptoms (weight gain, hair falling out, shaky, bad reaction to the medication, etc.):

Today, I am (emotional state):

Today, I accomplished/am happy about:

Today, I had the following stresses/things happen that upset me and/or my health:

FOOD LOG

(Write down what the food or drink was and how much of it you had)

For breakfast, I ate/drank:

For lunch, I ate/drank:

For dinner, I ate/drank:

For snacks, I ate/drank:

What did I do today that was good for my health and happiness?

What did I do today that could have been better for me?

What can I do differently tomorrow to make my day even more healthful?

Quantifying everything helps you gauge when things begin to improve, and it also helps you communicate with your doctor or other health professional when you present certain things to him or her in an easily translatable format.

Analyze your health journal

Once you have written in your health journal for several days, you can look back on what you've done and how you've felt and begin to identify good and bad cycles. Find a time when you felt good and happy. Thread through the circumstances around that time to see what support or other environmental factors led you to it. Did you exercise discipline and pass up dessert, feeling good about yourself and your willpower afterward? Did you make an effort with your appearance and reap uplifting compliments as a result? Did you take time to meditate and/or pray, clearing your mind of distractions and negative influences so that you could make the most of your quiet contemplation? Did that make you feel more in control of your health and life?

Also identify times when you fell short of helping yourself. Instead of passing up dessert, did the day's frustrations over your health and lack of energy make you shrug off weight concerns and eat a whole bag of cookies? And did you feel worse when you stood on your bathroom scale and discovered you'd gained more weight? Did someone's insensitive comment about your listlessness spur you to go into a frenzy of activity, only to make you more exhausted? When you thought about what you'd done, did you feel as though you were punishing yourself by trying to "show them," in spite of your physical constraints?

When you've identified the cycles in your life, both good and bad, you can begin to do something about what's harming you and do more of what's good for you. For example, if you tend to overeat or binge on something non-nutritional when you're angry, find a substitute activity that you can do instead (clean out a drawer, take a walk, talk out your emotions with a trusted friend). Before you begin eating anything, ask yourself if you really need the ribs, potato chips, or candy. Is what you're reaching for going to help you in terms of nutrition or fuel for your body?

If a friend's comments dig at your vulnerable, weakened self, approach him or her with the facts about your illness. From this position of helpful authority and strength, suggest ways that you can maintain your friendship on a more positive footing, given what you can and cannot do because of hypothyroidism. Be willing to be a friend as much as you want to have a friend.

Friends and family can be wonderful sources for perspective and suggestions. If you share with them your struggles, you could forge stronger ties with them and discover solutions to breaking your cycles. Perhaps, for example, a friend of yours suffers from low self-esteem, too. Suggest that you pool your resources and collections of cosmetics and do makeovers on one another, encouraging each other to maintain efforts to keep up appearances even after the "spa day" is over. Go shopping with one another, or just sit and talk openly about your feelings. Encourage one another. Don't be afraid to talk about spiritual matters, and how valuable you each are to the world around you, as well as to each other.

Men who feel dragged down by hypothyroidism can also rely on friends and family to lift them up through engaging in activities that require less energy but can foster strong moral support and camaraderie. For example, if you don't have the energy to do justice to a pickup game of basketball, join a bowling league, or take up golf and play nine holes instead of eighteen. In a world where men are supposed to never stop being active, defy convention and take time out to meditate and/or pray, refining your spirit and renewing your soul. If you practice prayer, consider joining a faith community where there is a strong presence of like-minded men and become involved with their activities. Remaining productive physically, mentally, and spiritually will make you more able to withstand the challenges of your illness *and* daily life.

Be proactive instead of reactive

One of the greatest trials in living with a chronic illness is finding the right level and kind of productivity. Sometimes, you have to substitute activities for ones you no longer have the physical ability to do. Other times, your perspective changes as you contemplate life from the angle of being chronically ill. Other times, you might think that the cycles you are in are enabling you to be productive when, in reality, they are doing you harm.

If you get caught up in negative cycles, you can dull your ability to be proactive about your health and other aspects of your life. As you review your health journal, highlight the times when you *reacted to* a situation or feeling instead of *taking charge* of it. Were there times when you felt so tired, so frustrated, so worthless that you just let the situation "be," enduring complaints and criticisms or allowing yourself to be dragged to events or to participate in activities that you were nowhere near up for? Or, did you give in to cravings because you couldn't imagine yourself saying no?

Create in your mind alternatives to these times, but don't be judgmental about them. For example, instead of saying, "I should have said no," write a script for yourself where you decline to participate or where you disengage yourself from a negative situation. If you have a hard time refusing a craving, substitute the thing you think you want with something that is more healthful (an apple instead of chocolate chip cookies, for instance, or working on an old car instead of going to the swap meet and overspending).

The next time you find yourself getting "trapped," take a deep breath, giving yourself time to recall your script and *use it* to enable yourself to be proactive and to take better care of yourself. Clue your family and friends into what you are trying to do and let them help you resist negative cycles by talking you through your actions and thoughts. Allow them to intervene at certain times, especially when you are feeling particularly weak. Consult with a psychologist, psychiatrist, or counselor about other ways that you can work against your urge to splurge. And don't forget to find good ways to reward yourself when you do break those negative cycles—you deserve it!

The benefits of the health journal

As you work through your health journal, you will discover ways that you can make your life easier without sacrificing your well-being. Being able to do this is a significant step in taking charge of your life and your illness. As your medication takes hold and you feel physically stronger, it will be easier to break the negative cycles and replace them with positive, healthful ones that will help you become even healthier and even more able to meet life's many challenges. As you succeed in turning your bad habits around, you will gain tremendous self-assurance and your courage will strengthen. And along the way, you will get to know many other people who can help guide you, as you will see in the next section.

IN A SENTENCE:

> *Identify cycles that lead you to do things that aren't good for you and take positive steps to move yourself toward better activities, thoughts, and health habits.*

learning

Needing and Finding Support

ON THE DAY you were diagnosed, your doctor probably told you when you need to return for a follow-up visit. Usually, this takes place a month or two from the day you began your medication. This is because it takes a while for the supplemental hormone to become fully integrated into your system. But between your first and next doctor's appointment, time doesn't stand still. There are a lot of things you wonder about regarding your condition and its treatment, and through your reading and conversation with others you will have even more questions. Your emotional state might be difficult to handle by yourself or even with your trusted family and friends.

There are people to whom you can turn for answers, and there are groups that provide information and support for hypothyroid patients. Starting with your medical team, you can rest assured that you are not alone.

Endocrinologists

The medical specialists who treat endocrine problems are **endocrinologists**. Besides thyroid function, they treat diabetes, reproductive hormonal problems, and other hormone-related syndromes and diseases. Some thyroid patients prefer that their endocrinologist be their main medical support for treating thyroid cancer, although **oncologists** often get involved, too.

An endocrinologist spends several extra years after medical school doing clinical work and residency in endocrinology. You might notice that some endocrinologists have "F.A.C.E." after their names. This is a professional designation indicating that the physician is a Fellow of the American Association of Clinical Endocrinologists (AACE). Some endocrinologists provide their specialty services as part of a group of doctors. Others maintain their own offices and patient base. There are few endocrinologists who specialize in thyroid disorders; many prefer to specialize in diabetes or reproductive endocrinology. But there are also thyroidologists, and once you find one, you will be in very good hands.

There are several ways to find an endocrinologist. Referrals from your doctor or fellow thyroid patients is a great way to get a personal opinion of the doctor and his or her way of approaching hypothyroidism. The AACE is an excellent place to go to find an endocrinologist in your area; their Web site is www.aace.org. The American Thyroid Association, or ATA (*www.thyroid.org*), is another good source to contact if you want to find an endocrinologist who specializes in thyroid disorders, as is the Thyroid Foundation of America (TFA) (*www.allthyroid.org.*)

Internal medicine specialist/general practitioner/family physician

An internal medicine physician has focused training and specializes in treating internal infections, diseases, and conditions such as hypothyroidism. Because he or she can treat other problems besides hypothyroidism, an internal medicine specialist can conduct tests and make diagnoses based upon your total health picture. Some internal medicine specialists might even conduct a woman's regular pap smear. General practitioners and family physicians also treat a wide range of illnesses and conditions in their practices. With them, too, you could have all of your examinations and tests for your thyroid and other health concerns.

There is always a trade-off between the convenience of having a "one-stop" doctor and getting specific care for your hypothyroidism. Some general practitioners are more likely to regard thyroid problems as "by the numbers" ailments and treat you accordingly. If you can find a physician who keeps up with the latest developments in endocrinology and, specifically, thyroidology, you are likely to get better treatment for your hypothyroidism. If your doctor is less well informed about thyroid issues, you can still go to him or her for other health matters, but find an endocrinologist for the specific treatment of hypothyroidism.

Another mark of a good general practitioner is if he or she refers you to a thyroid specialist. "So many medical offices and clinics are set up to tip the doctors to thyroid problems via the panel of blood tests that they run," says thyroidologist Elliot G. Levy, M.D. "A good doctor refers the patient to an endocrinologist."

Other medical professionals

Sometimes you might want to consult another specialist besides your doctor for symptoms that arise from your hypothyroidism. For example, if you need help coping with the emotional effects of hypothyroidism, you might want to speak with a **psychiatrist,** a medical doctor who specializes in mental health and who can prescribe medication. Other specialists who are not medical doctors but who might specialize in working with chronically ill patients are **psychologists** or **counselors. Licensed clinical social workers** and **clergypersons** sometimes counsel patients, too, but if you choose to go to one, make sure he or she is familiar with the issues related to coping with a chronic illness.

A **nutritionist** can help you understand issues related to weight gain and food. A **registered dietician** can help you do that, too. Your doctor should be able to provide you with referrals. Be careful of the "counseling" conducted at commercial weight loss centers; some might provide solid advice about managing your weight, but they might have no *medical* knowledge about hypothyroidism or the medication you are taking. The same is true of health food store workers and dietary supplement salespeople.

Pulmonologists treat disorders of the lungs, and **allergists** treat allergies and asthma. If you have asthma and feel that it might be exacerbated by your hypothyroidism (which does happen), an allergist can work with your endocrinologist or general practitioner to develop a regimen of allergy/asthma medications and ways to cope better while waiting for your hypothyroidism to stabilize. A **hemotologist,** a specialist in blood disorders and tests, can help you interpret your blood work results and suggest other tests that might shed light on your overall health picture.

You should get your eyes checked by an **ophthalmologist** at least once a year. Ophthalmologists are medical doctors who specialize in the eyes and can prescribe medication, and identify any optic complications from hypothyroidism. Thyroid eye disease is generally only found in people who are hyperthyroid, but when it occurs in hypothyroid patients, it requires competent medical care. **Optometrists** can examine your eyes for glaucoma and general functioning. **Opticians** make your eyeglasses from the prescription given by your ophthalmologist.

A **gynecologist** can perform a woman's regular pelvic and breast examination, as well as work with her endocrinologist or general practitioner to manage issues regarding fertility and PMS. There are also physicians who specialize in fertility, and you can usually get a referral to one from your gynecologist or general practitioner.

Alternative healthcare practitioners

Many hypothyroid patients are interested in combining their "traditional," Western-based medicinal treatments with holistic or alternative therapies. There is no herbal or alternative medication that can be used as a substitute for natural or synthetic thyroid hormone, but there are alternative treatments that can help relieve some of the lingering symptoms brought on by hypothyroidism. These are covered at length in Month 4.

Patient organizations

Managing a chronic illness can become very isolating, especially if you don't have much energy or are depressed. Finding a patient organization that provides information, support, and contact with others suffering as you do can make your life with hypothyroidism much less lonely. There are several such organizations, some of which have local chapters. Here's an overview of some of them, and you can find detailed contact information in the Resources section of this book.

○ **The American Thyroid Association.** This is the North American professional association for physicians and researchers specializing in the thyroid gland. The ATA offers some patient-oriented services, including referrals to ATA member physicians, publications on the

How to Select, Manage, and Communicate With Your Healthcare Professional

SOMETIMES, your medical insurance plan will dictate how much leeway you have in selecting the individuals responsible for providing you with healthcare. Even in those cases, you should always feel as though you are being given a high standard of attention and professional care. Here are some tips for ensuring that this happens:

Before or at your first doctor's visit, find out as much about your physician as possible. Ask about the doctor's training, expertise in treating thyroid disease, and philosophy toward treating the patient. Also find out about his or her availability after-hours, in case of emergency.

Next, observe your doctor's office. Was it clean? Well managed? Friendly? Overcrowded? Disorganized? Does the doctor and his or her staff respect your privacy; for example, do they close the door to allow you to get into your gown when they perform their examinations?

Take stock of your feelings in relation to your doctor and his or her office. How comfortable are you there? Do you genuinely trust this doctor and his or her staff with your healthcare?

Once you have selected your doctor, an important factor in maintaining a good patient/doctor relationship is clear, responsive communication. This is a two-way street. Your doctor should be a good listener, compassionate toward your fears and symptoms, but gently secure in his or her ability to treat them. You need to be willing to listen to your doctor, too, even if you don't like what he or she says (for example, if he or she tells you that you need to lose weight).

To help promote good communication, you should go to your appointments completely prepared. It will help if you write a "medical resume" and update it regularly. This should include:

Lists of your past ailments and/or surgeries, including dates and types of treatments you received for them.

Allergies to medications, environmental substances, and/or foods.

Medications you are now taking, for how long, and dosages. Include over-the-counter medications and herbs or other homeopathic substances.

Your current symptoms and complaints, as well as one or two key questions that you need answers to.

Always take a copy of this resume with you when you see a doctor for the first time. It will save you from having to repeat writing all your personal information with each new physician. Take two copies of your list of current medications and symptoms/questions with you to each subsequent visit. Use one for your reference (and write down on it what the doctor says in reply) and give one to your physician for his or her records.

Before you leave your doctor's office, make sure you understand what he or she said about changing or altering your medication or other treatment information. Know when you need to return for a follow-up visit. If you are having blood tests or other diagnostic tests run, know when you will get the results back and how these will be communicated to you (do you need to call your doctor or will your doctor or his or her office call you?). Also make sure you know if you need to fast beforehand or take any other pre-test action, or if you will be partially sedated and will need assistance getting home afterward.

major thyroid diseases, recommended books on thyroid disease, and public health statements on issues of importance to thyroid patients. On its Web site, you will find links to other thyroid patient organizations. The ATA also hosts the annual American Thyroid Association International convention where thyroid specialists from around the world meet to talk about recent research and developments in their fields of specialization. Concurrent with this convention are meetings of other thyroid patients' support organizations and press conferences to raise awareness in the general public about thyroid issues. The address is *www.thyroid.org*.

○ **The Thyroid Society** has been folded into the American Thyroid Association, but its Web site is still accessible and offers good basic information for patient education: *www.the-thyroid-society.org*.

○ **The Thyroid Foundation of America** was founded and is run *by* thyroid patients *for* thyroid patients. It encompasses all the thyroid disorders, including thyroid cancer, Graves' disease, and hypothyroidism. It offers information on thyroid disease and referrals to physicians in your area, opportunities for local patient support

When You and Your Doctor Don't Get Along

YOUR doctor need not become your best friend, but he or she should be willing to take your health seriously. Lisa Waldman, licensed clinical social worker and patient educator, says, "If you're getting symptom resolution and making progress, you might decide to stay with a doctor who doesn't have a great demeanor. You need someone who knows medicine, not just someone who's pleasant to be around. You don't want to compromise your health. But, if you're not getting satisfaction in terms of your health, you may need to consider making a change."

Areas where you might want to, or have to compromise to get the best healthcare are:

○ Distance. You might have to travel a bit farther to be seen by the right doctor.

○ Cost. You might have to pay more out-of-pocket for the proper healthcare.

○ Appointment times. Sometimes the best doctors are the busiest; you might have to wait awhile to be seen, but it is probably worth the wait.

"Once you determine that you have selected the doctor who is best for your health," says Waldman, "you can consider working toward improved communication by using a technique called diplomatic assertiveness." You will read more about diplomatic assertiveness and why it is such an important coping skill in Month 4.

groups, and other thyroid organizations. Its Web site is *www. allthyroid.org*.

○ **American Association of Clinical Endocrinologists** provides patient information of a technical nature and has a very informative Web site specific to thyroid disease at www.thyroidmanager.org. Their address is *www.aace.org*.

○ **National Graves' Disease Foundation.** If you started out with Graves' disease, this organization can provide you with information about coping with the change from being hyper- to hypothyroid. Its Web site is *www.ngdf.org*.

○ **ThyCa: Thyroid Cancer Survivors' Association.** This organization offers support, information, and useful links for people who are suffering or have suffered from thyroid cancer. It also has an area for posting jokes, some of which are hilarious! Its Web site is *www.thyca.org*.

○ **National Alopecia Areata Foundation.** This organization offers information and support to people suffering from one of the three forms of alopecia areata (areata, totalis, or universalis). Their Web site is: *www.naaf.org*.

○ The manufacturers of thyroid medications have medication/disease-focused Web sites and specific areas on their corporate Web sites devoted to information about their products and thyroid disease. Some also have toll-free hotlines that patients can call for further information. Many also offer Patient Assistance Programs that assist people with obtaining medication if they cannot otherwise afford it. You can find a list of these located in the Resources section of this book.

"Outside the Box" support

Other organizations that aren't necessarily tied to thyroid disease might be able to help with your specific needs, too. Consider joining Overeaters Anonymous if overeating is a problem. Women's support groups can help you manage your familial and personal issues. Therapy support groups can be helpful, too, and some people feel more comfortable talking in a group than one-on-one with a counselor.

Friends and family

When you are seeking support for your condition, do not forget those closest to you: your friends and family. They might not understand what you are going through, but sometimes just their presence can take the edge off of your discomfort and anxiety. Help them to learn more about your condition, and encourage them to talk with other patients or loved ones, if that will enable them to be more comfortable about hypothyroidism.

As you educate your loved ones, remember to be a friend to them, too. Having a chronic illness can make you more self-centered than you normally would be, and it might take extra effort to reach out to others. But you will find that by listening to *their* problems and celebrating *their* triumphs, you will feel less lonely and more fulfilled.

Some of the concrete ways to include your loved ones in your health-care are:

○ Inviting them to come to a doctor's appointment with you, or to make their own appointment with your physician, so that they can ask and get answers to their specific questions and concerns;

○ Encouraging them to continue their thyroid education by sharing your newsletters, books, and other information with them;

○ Including them in your patient support groups (if appropriate) or helping them find a support group specifically for loved ones of hypothyroidism sufferers.

○ Helping them to maintain their own health and identity, making sure that they are able to continue their activities and interests.

Faith and spirit

With a chronic illness taking hold of you inside and many changes and uncertainties in the world around you, the role of faith and spirit may take on greater importance for you. If you are a believer before you become ill, your purpose in the world and the reason for your illness are folded up in the sense that you matter to something beyond your daily routine. If you question the existence of God, or did not believe before your diagnosis, sometimes facing a chronic illness can spur you on to explore more spiritual possibilities in living. And if you are angry with God, wondering why He allowed you to get sick, you are still carrying on an inner dialogue that goes beyond yourself and your health problems.

In this first week since your diagnosis, take extra time out of each day to sit quietly and take stock of all that has happened to you and how you feel emotionally and spiritually. Look beyond the obvious fatigue and other symptoms to examine the root of your very being. Are you afraid? Anxious? Angry? Shaken? Are you disappointed with God?

As you delve deeper into yourself, you might be surprised that there is good mixed in with the bad. Perhaps you are relieved at your diagnosis, and you lift up a small prayer of "thanks" for the insight of your doctors and the possibility of medicine to treat your condition. Or, you might be joyful that your hypothyroidism is not a terminal illness. By taking more time for introspection, you are also likely to learn more about yourself and your place in the world. In doing so, you will no doubt find more treasures to uncover, and happiness, too.

As you sit in the quiet, make a specific commitment to get to know your inner self and the spirit that is within you and learn to listen better. Let the balm of quiet run over you like cool water and let your spirit relax with the truth that you will take more time from now on to nurture this core, this center within you. Revel in the uniqueness of your inner spirit and prayer life and/or meditation, if you engage in these practices. There is no one else like you, inside and out. Look upon your illness as a way to further establish your individualism and encourage your talents and dreams.

Beyond your quiet time, you also might like to share some of your insight with a faith community. Their spiritual support and prayers can be a tremendous help for you as you continue to grapple with all that hypothyroidism means in your life now and in the years to come. By doing this, you will nurture your spiritual side and be able to benefit from its growing strength as you face the challenges and the joys of the days ahead.

IN A SENTENCE:

> *There are many organizations and people who can support you as you face the challenges of hypothyroidism, and you can find support spiritually, too, through meditation and/or prayer.*

DAY **6**

living

Stress and Hypothyroidism

HOW YOU cope with stress can make a huge difference in how quickly your body rebounds from the effects of hypothyroidism, as well as how healthy you are able to stay overall. The medical community has still not definitively said that there is a correlation between autoimmune illnesses and stress; we cannot say for sure that stress *causes* hypothyroidism. But there seems to be a growing body of medical wisdom that suggests that illness, particularly autoimmune illness, can be triggered by stressful events. And just from the way stress impacts those of us who do suffer from chronic illness, we can be sure that the pressure and physical effects of stress are not nurturing for our spirits, emotional states, and, ultimately, our physical well-being.

Unfortunately, there are some stresses over which we have no control. But there are things you can do to better cope with them. The sooner you develop excellent coping skills the better off you will be when inevitable stressful events occur. And the best place to start is by gaining insight into what stress is and how it affects you and the world around you.

Identifying stress

As it relates to our lives, stress is something that creates in us a sense of tension, agitation, and/or anxiety. Through my own experience of being a patient and trying to lessen stress in my life, I've come to learn that there are basically two kinds of stress: *anticipated* stress and *unexpected* stress. That is, some of life's stresses occur unexpectedly, but some of them can be anticipated and either managed or alleviated completely. Anticipated stress occurs when you put yourself in a situation that you know has the potential of being stressful, but you do it anyway. Examples of this are:

○ Choosing to go to the supermarket at the busiest times, when the lines are longest and the parking lot is full.
○ Agreeing to go out with a friend who saps your energy and always manages to pay less than what you do when you split the bill for dinner.
○ Scheduling so many things on your "day off" that you are more tense at the end of the day than when you began.
○ Overspending and, as a result, not having enough money at the end of the month for necessary expenses.
○ Ignoring your health or symptoms and waiting to seek treatment until your condition is critical.
○ Taking on so many responsibilities at work that you do not do justice to any one of them.

With anticipated stress, you *know* before you proceed that the situation you're moving into will be stressful. You *dread* it, you *procrastinate,* you find every way you can to *get out* of it. And once you are in the midst of it, you feel an overwhelming sense of wanting to escape as quickly as you can.

Another aspect of your reaction to anticipated stress, especially to things that you *choose* to do, is a physical reaction that contributes to your overall sense of poor health. When you move into a stressful situation, the following physical things might happen:

○ Your muscles *tighten* in your stomach, shoulders, or neck;
○ Your hands feel *clammy* and *moist*;
○ Your mouth gets *dry*;

○ You forget to *breathe;*

○ You might *shiver* or *shake* or *fidget* with a paper clip, pencil, rubber band, the sleeve of your sweater, or the telephone cord.

○ Your *pulse* might race and your eyelids might *flutter.*

○ You might tug at the hair on your head, eyebrows, or back of your hand.

Anticipated stress can affect you before it occurs, too, especially since you *know* that it is coming up. Oftentimes your sleep patterns will be disrupted the night before a day you know will be stressful. You might lose your appetite, and you might also feel "heavier," as though you don't want to move forward into the stressful event.

Many times, when the event or activity that precipitates your reactions to anticipated stress is over, you return to feeling calm, and the physical and emotional effects the stress had upon you fade away. Still, it is important to realize that you have had a stress event, and your body, which has just been through the wringer, needs time to rest.

Although healthy people also feel the effects of anticipated stress, when you are faced with it *and* a chronic illness, you run the risk of exacerbating your symptoms or developing new ones. Also, if you open yourself up to too much stress on a regular basis, the physical effects of it will not as readily dissipate, leaving you in a near-constant state of stress.

Of course, we cannot live our lives without stress. There will always be times when we can't avoid Christmas shopping on the weekend before the holiday, sharing a meal with someone who "rubs us the wrong way," or feeling "crunch time" on the job. But the more we control the anticipated stresses in our lives, the better off we will feel and, thus, the better off we'll be.

Getting control of anticipated stress

Using your health journal and observational skills, identify the ways in which you create stressful situations or the times you leave yourself open to stresses in your life. Remember, this is not the time to be a *victim* of stress, but rather it is a time to be honest and see where you might be allowing extra stress into your life.

Identify which anticipated stresses you tend to come in contact with repeatedly. Each month, do you have to rush over to the pharmacy just before it closes to get your next month's supply of meds? Do you have a habit of eating sugary foods just before bed and, as a result, toss and turn uncomfortably for hours into the night? Examine your relationships with others, too, and look for the telltale effects of anticipated stress when you talk to them on the telephone, spend time with them, or think about them.

The actions and events that bring about repeated, anticipated stresses are those that you should do something about first. As you have when you try to break negative cycles, develop a "script" for yourself that shows you a way to move away from the stresses. Recognize that you do have a chronic illness and you need to be mindful of the limitations imposed on you by it. Allow time for your "down" days, and schedule picking up your meds or other regular tasks a few days ahead of time so that, if you are laid up in bed, you won't feel stressed about missing essential activities.

Unexpected stress

The kind of stress that I have found more difficult to deal with in my life is *unexpected stress*. This includes the loss of a loved one, a move, a job change, a divorce, in short, anything that uproots a significant part of life and, sometimes, brings deep emotional pain.

I felt a horribly powerful pain one year after I was diagnosed with lupus. My brother, my only sibling, died very unexpectedly. The news shocked me to my soul. The aftermath was just as shocking, as I was caught up in all that goes into saying good-bye to someone very beloved. The stress sent my lupus into even more of a flare, and for months, I was rocked by sadness, anger, terrible dreams, and bitter, unanswered questions.

How did I cope with having a severe chronic illness *and* a traumatic life event all at once? Well, I don't think there's any "secret" formula. Getting onto an even keel after such a trial isn't something that happens overnight, nor is it something that heals by following a prescribed number of "steps." But here are some things that I found very helpful:

- ○ **Let your doctor know what's happened.** Immediately upon hearing about my brother's death, I called my loved ones and my doctor. I relied on all of them for moral support, and asked my doctor specifically if there was anything I could do so that the stress didn't overwhelm me. My doctor continued to monitor my health condition and offered compassionate support that helped tremendously in the days and months to follow. If you are not comfortable talking with your doctor about important and painful events in your life that might affect your health, you should probably think about finding another doctor.

O **Let others help.** From the day I got the news, I let friends do things for me. Bring me dinner. Talk on the phone. Be there for me. I allowed their abilities to take charge of my life, disabled as it was, and I can't begin to say how much that meant to me, emotionally, spiritually, and physically.

O **Continue to take care of your health.** I *continued* to take my medication and in other ways tried to take care of my health as best I could. Letting my healthcare slip wouldn't have done anyone any good, least of all myself. (I was less successful in remembering to feed my fish regularly, so I had to post notes to myself on the front door every day so I didn't forget!)

O **Express your grief.** Expressing grief was difficult because I have Sjogren's syndrome, an autoimmune syndrome that affects the tear ducts, saliva glands, and other moisture-producing glands in the body. Sometimes, I couldn't cry at all; my eyes would make no tears. Other times, only one eye would cry. I found other ways to express my grief, sometimes just moving around my apartment, or staring out the window.

O **Prayer.** Throughout the days and months following my brother's death, my faith was central. I prayed, listened to inspirational music, went to church, and gave myself plenty of time for God's healing to work.

O **Gain knowledge about what you're going through.** After the memorial service and some time had passed, I went to a local church's bereavement program. At first, I thought it was going to be depressing. But soon I learned so much about grieving that I found it very uplifting. *Gaining knowledge* about what you are going through is extremely empowering—and there's a lot about grieving that we don't begin to know until we go through it.

○ **Be nice to yourself.** I didn't go overboard, but I did take time and effort to be nice to myself and to shield myself from unnecessary stressful events that could have exacerbated my fragile emotional and physical state.

○ **Focus on accepting what you're going through.** As heart-wrenching as it was, there was no doubt about what had happened. I'd lost my only sibling, my beloved brother. I accepted my emotional state and gave it time, lots of time, to work through. This is so very important; any unexpected stress is going to cause lingering effects, and you have to be prepared to give it time.

○ **Recognize the signs of depression and address them.** Severe stress and crises can be so overwhelming that they bring on depression. Be aware that this might happen and accept it if it does; there is no shame in depression, and there are many things that you can do to help yourself recover from it.

○ **Do the best you can.** We don't get a grade for how well we cope with crises. We don't "fail" or "pass with honors." We can't hold ourselves up to someone else, trying to "live up to" their standards. We can only strive to do the best that we can with the circumstances we are given. Be honest with yourself as you cope. Recognize that you aren't going to do everything perfectly, nor will everything turn out "just right." But do the best that you can, with love and patience, and you will get through the darkest trial.

World events and you

Today more than ever, we live in uncertain times. Besides the personal crises that might affect us, there are forces beyond our control in the world around us. The stress that that knowledge gives us, and the added stress of natural and unnatural disasters that occur, can oppress our spirits and aggravate our chronic health conditions. Besides relying on the coping mechanisms I've already mentioned, taking precautions to make your surroundings as safe as possible will help you feel more in control of your world. If you live in an earthquake-prone area, having an earthquake kit and a plan of communication with loved ones is essential. Knowing where the fire escapes are in your workplace is also important. Making sure your medication is close at hand in case you have to take refuge in your basement because of a tornado warning is vital to keeping your peace of mind intact as it regards your health.

Make a list of the things you need to do to feel prepared in case of emergency. Don't forget to prepare your children and yourself emotionally, too. Emergencies do happen. We all have to live with them. But, as with anticipated stresses, we can do many things to ease our worries and go about our daily lives with a good sense of preparedness.

"Good stress"

I once heard a doctor say that "stress is stress, whether it comes from good or bad things or events." In fact, the physical reactions to good stress—wonderful surprises, the birth of a child, a marriage proposal— are often identical to those we might have when bad things happen. The pulse quickens, the mouth gets dry, the body trembles. I certainly become more forgetful!

Good things *are* more desirable than bad, and we welcome them willingly into our lives. But even in the best of times, we can't forget to take care of our health and give ourselves a little extra rest, a little extra consideration, so that we can maintain our quality of life and take full advantage of the good things that come our way.

Lessons learned

Stress will never go away completely. The coping strategies you develop in the midst of crisis are those that you can call upon again and again. When I was diagnosed with Hashimoto's thyroiditis, my aunt was in the end stage of pancreatic cancer. This was very traumatic for our whole extended family, and was compounded, for me, by being so far away from my loved ones. I called upon my support system, my faith, and the other tools I'd developed in other difficult times to cope with and, I hope, be of support to her and other family members in my aunt's last days.

As you take stock of how weak you feel physically, and how hard you are trying to struggle through each day with the symptoms of hypothyroidism, you might say, "I can't do this. I just couldn't cope with anything more." But the reality is, you can. And you will, if you give yourself the chance to learn about stress and your reaction to it, find your strengths, and make good use of them as well as the support network that you already have and will further develop as the days go by.

IN A SENTENCE:

> *Stress can have physical and emotional effects on your health and well-being, but by identifying and taking control of some of the stress in your life, you can greatly lessen the negative effect it has on you.*

learning

The Mind/Body Thyroid Connection: Depression

WHETHER IT rises from stress, traumatic life events, crises, or an illness, depression can be mild or life-altering, a faint cloud on the horizon or a full-blown storm. When you are depressed, you might feel particularly helpless or as though you've failed in some kind of "life test." This can further exacerbate your feelings of low self-worth and can actually worsen your depression.

No one, hypothyroid or not, is immune to being depressed at some point in his or her life. But depression in someone who is hypothyroid can carry its own unique circumstances

Lidia Q. says, "I never went to get help for the depression, which was a stupid thing. I should have told the doctor, but in my family, that wasn't done."

Lisa Waldman, licensed clinical social worker and patient educator, says, "Depression needs to be addressed inside and outside the patient. That is, if the depression is biologically based—brought on by a chemical or hormonal imbalance related to an illness or medication—it should be treated medically, just like any other symptom. This type of depression can be effectively treated with medication.

"If life's stressors or a patient's own attitudes and behaviors are causing depression, then other methods of coping should be undertaken and psychological counseling may be considered. Quite often, both biological and personal factors play a role in depression. In this case, medication along with counseling will be most helpful. Unfortunately, some people still feel a stigma about taking antidepressant medication or getting other psychological help. But it is really important to seek these options."

Also important is understanding that depression is something that a lot of hypothyroid patients suffer from, for a variety of reasons. There is nothing wrong with being depressed; you haven't failed and you aren't worthless. Above all, depression is something that can be identified and treated—and you *can* feel better.

Identifying and quantifying depression

According to the Mayo Clinic, there are two "hallmarks" of depression: Loss of interest in normal daily activities, and a depressed mood (sadness, helplessness, hopelessness, crying spells).[1] These can certainly be manifested in hypothyroid patients; if you are severely fatigued, you can lose interest in your daily life, and your mood can also become depressed because of your health condition and the strain it puts on your life. When some hypothyroid patients are depressed, they cry readily. Others withdraw from the world around them.

There are other more physical indications of depression and symptoms that might mimic depression but that are related to physical problems such as hypothyroidism. These include loss of appetite, muscular pain, and "brain fog."

In order to identify the root of your symptoms and depression, you should have your doctor perform a physical examination and go over certain questions with you. These questions will give you and your doctor insight into psychological manifestations of depression and include:

- Have you had trouble sleeping on a regular basis?
- Have you experienced any significant weight loss or gain?
- Do you feel worthless? Do you have thoughts of death, dying, or suicide?

○ Do you have trouble concentrating or making decisions? Are you more forgetful than you usually are?

○ Do you cry easily? Are you frequently edgy, nervous, or moody?

Catastrophic life events and stress, such as the loss of a spouse, child, or other loved one; an accident; the loss of a job, or divorce, can precipitate depression. Deep dissatisfaction with a part or all of your life can influence it, too. During the course of your examination, you should share these things with your doctor and, if you can, give a quantifiable number to the extent to which these things figure in your life.

There can be chemical reasons for depression, as well, such as a lack of **serotonin** and/or thyroid or other hormones. Sometimes, blood tests can reveal if there are any deficiencies here.

When you have the data from your physical examination and answers to the above questions, your doctor will be better able to determine which part of your symptoms might be related to physical health issues, which are more psychological in nature, and which might overlap. He or she will then be able to suggest a course of action to bring both your body and mind into better balance. There is every cause for hope at this point: In taking action to look after your health and well-being, you are being strong and resilient!

How does thyroid hormone influence mood?

Sometimes, signs of depression dissipate as you get farther into your supplemental thyroid hormone replacement therapy. As your medication begins to work and your thyroid hormone levels improve, you might feel as if a cloud is lifting from you and the sunshine is pouring through. This could be due to a number of factors, among them that your body is receiving more metabolic hormone and is functioning more optimally. Better brain function can also bring an increase in your **serotonin** levels.

Serotonin is a brain chemical that plays a crucial role in regulating your mood. Because thyroid hormone regulates your metabolism, and your brain needs adequate amounts of thyroid hormone to function properly, sometimes hypothyroid patients become depressed. Many times, this depression lessens or lifts completely once adequate thyroid medication has a chance to work. Other times, patients need additional treatments in conjunction with their thyroid therapy to get back to feeling well in body and mind.

Sometimes, too, hypothyroid patients experience depression that is not a result of their thyroid condition, but rather is due to other causes. Exploring these with your doctor and seeking help can greatly improve your overall quality of life.

Psychologists and psychiatrists

Psychotherapy or counseling can be very effective to help you through the difficult, early days of diagnosis and treatment for depression. A trained counselor can assist you in identifying troubling issues concerning your health and other aspects of your life and can also help you to work out a game plan for coping with them. You need not look upon counseling as a long-term form of treatment; once your medication is adjusted appropriately, you might not need to see a counselor at all. But the extra support you get early on can give you more strength and hope as you get going.

A psychologist or marriage and family counselor (MFCC) can also guide you through your introspection and help you cope as you climb out of your depression. A psychiatrist can help you here, too, and can also prescribe additional medication, if you need more chemical assistance in overcoming your depression.

Sometimes, people who are grappling with depression also call upon their clergyperson or faith community for spiritual guidance. This, together with a vibrant meditation or prayer life, can help you reach insights about your life that are bright and new.

Medication for depression

If your doctor or psychiatrist recommends you take medication for your depression, do not look upon it as a stigma, but rather as an empowering step toward helping you gain control of your health. Medication, along with the other things you are doing to improve your health, might bring you more strength than you ever thought possible.

Among the classifications of medications used to treat depression are **selective serotonin reuptake inhibitors** (SSRIs). These elevate the amount of serotonin in your system and are often considered first to treat depression Examples of SSRIs are flouxetine (Prozac, Sarafem), paroxetine (Paxil), sertraline (Zoloft), and citalopram (Celexa).

Tricyclic and **tetracyclic antidepressants** work in a similar way to SSRIs, but by a different mechanism. Examples of tricyclic antidepressants are amitriptyline (Elavil, Endep), desipramine (Norpramin, Pertofrane), and protriptyline (Vivactil). Some tetracyclics are maprotiline (Ludiomil) and mirtazapine (Remeron). These are often used by doctors to treat moderate to severe depression.

If you take lithium, be sure to tell your doctor. Sometimes lithium can induce goiter and/or hypothyroidism. As with any medication, call your doctor immediately if you experience any adverse side effects.

Sometimes, it takes several weeks for you to feel the full effect of anti-depression medication. Also, it might take several tries before you find the medication that works well for you. This is because our body chemistries are unique, and we respond differently to these different medications.

When you start with any antidepression medication, ask both your physician and your pharmacist about side effects and how to gauge if and how much the medication is working. Also ask how you should time taking your antidepressant because it can sometimes interfere with your thyroid meds.

Check in with your doctor regularly, keeping your health journal each day so that you can carefully chart your physical reaction to the medication and how much your mood is affected by it. Be patient. Some of these medications work very subtly, and you won't realize they're working until you get farther down the road and are able to look back and see just how wonderfully far you've come.

Meditation or prayer

Can meditation or prayer cure depression? Those who believe in miracles would say, "Yes. With God, anything is possible." Skeptics, on the other hand, would say, "No way." For many people, miracles happen in far-off lands to complete strangers. You might not have considered miraculous healing until recently, when you were faced with having a chronic illness and became part of the medical system. Perhaps people you know have already told you that they would pray for your total healing. And you might have prayed for it, too, even though you doubt that such a thing could ever happen to you.

Between the belief in complete healing and atheism is a middle ground that many chronically ill sufferers enjoy. Even without scientific proof that faith healing happens, these people find comfort and encouragement in maintaining active spiritual lives. The peace and quiet of soul and heart that come from finding refuge from the stresses of the day can help soothe the deep wounds of disappointment and sadness that come from living with chronic illness. Time after time, when I conducted my interviews of hypo-thyroid patients, I heard of how prayer figured prominently into many of their "prescriptions for good health."

"I went through a lot of meditation. Prayer was natural to me, too," says Julie N., who went so long without a diagnosis that she developed deep depression. "I had a prayer that I set up in front of me on my desk that I read every morning, as often as I needed to, to get through the day."

"I keep a prayer journal," says Pamela G., "I can go back and see where things have been answered. It might seem like a small thing to do, but after a while, it becomes big." Prayer is important in my own life, and opens each day and closes each night. I don't feel disappointed that I haven't been cured of my illnesses, but I do feel peaceful as I rest in the calming, peace-ful center that is a place of retreat and prayer.

More doctors, such as Larry Dossey, M.D.[3], and Harold G. Koenig, M.D.[4], are exploring the effects of prayer on physical well-being and heal-ing. Some medical schools are also exploring the connection, even includ-ing a prayer and meditation component in their patient-care training.

In a state of quiet contemplation, heart rate, blood pressure, and other physical signs of depression and stress may become less problematic, enabling you to better equip yourself to face life's challenges. Also, prayer can lead you to accept your condition more readily, approaching it from a calm, patient position instead of the maelstrom that sometimes sweeps you up when you are faced head-on with the pain and challenges of hypo-thyroidism.

Prayer can take many forms, but is most effective when it helps the sup-plicant accept his or her situation and relationship with God.

"There are a lot of different prayers," says Frank Desiderio, C.S.P., pro-ducer of the Arts and Entertainment network's documentary on healing and prayer, "But the most effective one is, 'Thy will be done.'"

Getting to that point is calming and means that you accept your condi-tion and so can move on with more acceptance and resolve. This, in turn, can give you focused energy to tackle the challenges that life and your illness throw at you—and as hypothyroid patients, we need all the energy we can get!

Meditation, too, can help your body become centered on calm, peace, and healing. Sitting in a quiet place, and reflecting on your safety and relaxation, can bring you much pleasure and insight into yourself and your life in ways that you never even imagined.

One of the keys to meditating and/or praying most beneficially is to practice deep breathing. This age-old technique of allowing fresh air to "cleanse" your inner self from stresses and staleness and to release all that negative influence from your body is also an excellent way to help your body relax and your tension level to decrease. And the better you breathe, the more you will be able to benefit from your prayer and/or meditation sessions.

Where to begin?

There are four key components to getting the most from a breathing, meditation, or prayer regimen.

- ○ **A quiet, comfortable environment**. If you are thinking too much about where you are, or are physically uncomfortable or rattled by outside noises, you won't be able to relax. When you are ready to center yourself quietly, select a place where you will not be distracted. This might be a chapel, the beach, or a room of your own at home. If you are at home, take your telephone off the hook, or let the answering machine pick up your calls. If there are others around, such as family members, tell them that you do not want to be disturbed for a certain amount of time. Stick to this resolve to not be disturbed—at first, it might be difficult, but it is always helpful to learn when to say no.
- ○ **A focused mind and heart**. You might not have to work hard at meditating and/or praying, but you do need to get yourself into the right frame of mind to be open to the experience. Tell yourself that you will tackle your problems and other tasks after your quiet time. If you make the most of this time alone, you will probably find that you will be stronger when it comes to meeting outside challenges.

Use visualization to get yourself into the right "place" for your quiet time. Imagine yourself in your favorite vacation spot or other far-away place. Also, you might keep something simple and soothing at hand, such as a rosary or set of prayer beads, so that you can use your sense of touch to put you further into that position of contemplation. Another good object to focus on is a lit candle; the flicker of the flame can be very soothing.

○ **A comfortable physical position.** You don't have to try a pretzel-like yoga position in order to meditate or pray, nor do you need to fast beforehand. In fact, if you are straining your muscles or your stomach is growling from hunger, you are more likely to do harm to your quiet time and your physical self. Make sure that you are wearing comfortable clothing and can truly relax your body so that you don't focus on it throughout the time you've set aside for your spirit and heart.

○ **A regular meditation and/or prayer schedule.** Find a time of the day when you can have five, ten, or fifteen uninterrupted minutes in a quiet place and try to take just that much time each day. This can become your "oasis" in the midst of a hectic schedule and people who make demands on you, and you should treasure it just as you would the time you spend taking care of other aspects of your health.

You might choose to begin your meditation or prayer with something structured, such as a written prayer or book that contains focused meditations. There are also classes in different forms of meditation, many of which are based on Eastern religions and worship practices. Whichever way you choose, be sure that you are benefiting from the time you spend in quiet and contemplation. Sometimes, especially when the world seems to be spinning out of control around you, the simplest forms of prayer or meditation work best to calm you and help you find a solid center.

Faith communities

Another way to benefit from prayer and the support of others is to join a faith community and participate in its collective worship and prayer life. Finding the congregation that is right for you might take some time, but it

A Bit about Breathing

BREATHING is usually something we do automatically. However, when you couple more conscious, controlled breathing with your meditation or prayer, you can benefit from extra relaxation and focus. Here is one way to practice deep breathing as an adjunct to your reflective times:

Place your hand gently on the lowest area of your ribcage (where your diaphragm is, just above your abdomen). Breathe in through your nose, counting to three slowly. Feel your hand rise as you take in the air deeply with the assistance of your diaphragm. Count "one." Breathe out slowly through your mouth until all the air you've taken in has been expelled. As you prepare to take another breath, do an internal "check" of which muscles seem most relaxed and which still seem tense. Target the tense areas with your next breath, as if taking in the fresh air will cleanse these places of their stress. As you breathe out, imagine that you are sending all the tension out, too.

After you have breathed deeply two or three times, begin meditating and/or praying, breathing normally. If you feel yourself tensing, try your deep breathing again once or twice, focusing on letting your tension out. When you have finished praying and/or meditating, spend a few moments quietly, listening to your body breathe, and respond to your time of relaxation. You might find that you are so relaxed that you're ready to fall asleep! In fact, this breathing technique is something I use when I need to relax my tensed muscles and fibromyalgia symptoms before bedtime. It makes a huge difference!

will be worth it when you find a "spiritual home" that can be a natural extension of your own inner prayer work. Faith communities often pitch in tangibly when you are too ill to cook, run errands, or watch your children. And they can provide you with a place in which to be productive, especially if you're not able to work full-time outside the home; volunteer opportunities within a church, synagogue, or mosque are usually unlimited.

Examining attitude

Once you address your depression from a medical angle and your thyroid medication starts working, you might need to explore other more personality-driven aspects of your attitude to feel psychologically and spiritually better. One key here is to look at how you view the world and how you think.

"Thoughts influence the emotions," says Lisa Waldman. "If you have negative and pessimistic thoughts, your emotions might be negative, too. When evaluating your depression, ask yourself if you have a tendency to think negatively. Do you imagine the glass half empty instead of half full? Is this a way of viewing the world that began prior to your illness?"

Other traits to consider are:

○ Do you tend to think the worst or overreact to daily problems? ("My hand itches so I just know I'm going to develop a rash all over my body.")

○ Do you take the worst of a situation and generalize so that it becomes the standard for everything else? ("I know three people on thyroid hormone and they're not feeling better, so I won't, either.")

○ Do you think in "black and white?" That is, do you think things are either all good or all bad? ("I have hypothyroidism so my life is ruined.")

○ Do you believe in "all or nothing?" ("If I can't do all the housework today, what's the point in doing any of it?")

Improving your outlook might be as easy as doing things that you once found enjoyable, such as a hobby or sport. Other positive activities include doing things that make you laugh, spending time with people who care about you and your experience, and finding a new hobby or interest.

"If people are very consistent and disciplined, they can have a profound impact on their outlook and, thus, on their overall well-being," says Waldman. "Some people can do this on their own through affirmations, books, social support, and spiritual communities. Others don't have that kind of discipline and can benefit from counseling. Sometimes, too, there are deeper issues preventing positive coping, and by working with a psychotherapist, these can be resolved."

IN A SENTENCE:

> *Depression is common among hypothyroid patients and can be treated successfully by working with your medical team to address the physical aspect of it and taking time to take care of your inner self.*

Your Weight and Hypothyroidism: Myth and Fact

MANY HYPOTHYROID patients complain of weight gain before, during, and after they are diagnosed. For some, like me, the gain is only a few pounds, and is unwelcome, but hardly debilitating. For others, the pounds keep coming and the resulting gain can be fifty, a hundred, even two hundred–plus pounds of heaviness that can cause additional health problems of its own.

Having struggled with it myself, I knew that weight gain is one of the topics that we hypothyroid patients find especially important. So much of our self-esteem is wrapped up in how we look, and so much of how we look is dependent upon our weight. Also, much of our overall health is dependent upon how fit we are and how little extra weight and stress is put on our internal organs (heart, lungs, kidneys, pancreas) and joints (especially the knees and hips). But just what is the truth about gaining weight due to hypothyroidism? Is it inevitable? Permanent? Are we hypothyroid sufferers doomed to be "hypo-hippos" (I made that name up on a day when I was feeling particularly paunchy), or is there something we can do to gain control of our weight and thus improve our health and self-image?

In my research, I immediately found more information than was easily digestible (please pardon the pun) concerning this sensitive topic. In discussions with other hypothyroid patients, books, pamphlets, advertisements, and Internet Web sites, there were recommended diets, dietary supplements, herbs, "spices," and a myriad of other approaches to taking off extra pounds—and many of them were said to apply to hypothyroid-related, as well as overall weight gain. In fact, in some dietary supplements and weight-loss centers' programs, supplemental thyroid hormone, particularly T_3, is used as a weight-control drug, irregardless of whether the person it's given to needs it for thyroid purposes.

It became quite clear to me that I needed to get down to basics to make sense of it for myself and for you. Here are the guidelines that will form the basis for this discussion on weight and hypothyroidism:

○ Weight categories (underweight, normal weight, overweight, obesity) are those given by the National Institutes of Health for their **body mass index** (BMI) guidelines.

○ Weight gain that can be attributed strictly to hypothyroidism (that is, the absence of adequate thyroid hormone) is usually between 5 and 10 pounds.

○ Weight gain above that as a direct result of inadequate thyroid hormone comes from a variety of causes, including eating disorders, improper diet, and lack of exercise, which might be related to hypothyroidism, too, but not necessarily caused by it.

○ There is one clear fact about eating and weight gain: You have complete control over what you put in your body.

Body mass index and determining weight status

The National Institutes of Health, a government agency that conducts research and provides public and medical professional information on a wide range of health issues, has a Web site with a section devoted to the **body mass index**, or BMI (www.nhlbisupport.com/bmi). The BMI provides an easy way to categorize your particular weight situation, devoid of value judgments and personal perceptions. There, you will find an easy-to-use form that will calculate your BMI based on the height and weight that you input on the screen. Once you have your BMI, you can consult the categories that are listed to the left of the form to see if you are underweight (BMI of less than 18.5), normal weight (BMI of 18.5-24.9), overweight (BMI of 25-29.9), or obese (BMI of 30 or greater). The BMI table and the form pertain to men as well as women.

If you do not have access to the Internet, or you want to check your BMI quickly, consult the chart on page 95 that lists BMIs, with the four weight categories listed. As you can see by looking at the chart, there are ranges within each of the categories. This allows for a variety of body types at each height; if you are "big boned," for example, you might still be in the normal range, even if you weigh more than a friend of yours who is the same height.

Knowing your BMI will help you determine the extent of your weight problem (if you have one) and put your mind at ease if you are in the normal range. Of course, it is still important to exercise and eat healthfully—a bad diet can also cause cholesterol problems, as well as other health ailments. But sometimes it is good to see, in print, that our weight is on target, even if we have those days when we still "feel fat," or our weight fluctuates because of hypothyroidism or other reasons. This is particularly important for people who have gone from being hyperthyroid to hypothyroid, or for those who had their thyroid glands surgically removed and suddenly find themselves without adequate thyroid hormone.

Hypothyroidism and weight gain

There are several factors that contribute to hypothyroid patients gaining weight, especially before they begin thyroid hormone therapy. These factors range from the physiological to the psychological, and are almost all manageable, to some extent. In fact, several of the physicians whom I interviewed regarding weight gain and hypothyroidism said that, in their clinical experience, only between five to ten pounds of the weight gain experienced by the average hypothyroid patient is attributable directly to their lack of adequate thyroid hormone. Any more weight gain than that indicates other factors, such as dietary choices and lack of exercise, which may be partly related to a patient's response to being hypothyroid, but not due to the lack of thyroid hormone alone.

From Hyper- to Hypo-

I STARTED out with hyperthyroidism, and lived for nearly twenty years with the sometimes heady feeling that I could never gain weight. Oh, maybe at certain times of the month I'd gain a few pounds. But those were easily shed when my monthly cycle moved on. Now, however, I understand that my metabolism was behaving very differently than it does now that I am hypothyroid, and my mind-set was also different. Now I have to radically rethink my approach to weight, weight gain, and what I eat, adjusting my expectations to what is truly "normal," as opposed to what was truly "abnormal" when I was hyperthyroid. If you, too, have been hyperthyroid and are now hypothyroid, give yourself time to get to know your body all over again. Understand that you have to expect that you'll think you're heavy when, actually, you are "normal." Consult the BMI to find your weight category, and discuss your metabolism issues frankly with your doctor. Counseling, too, might help you readjust to this "new you," which is going to be with you for years to come.

Looking at the weight gain issue first from the perspective of hypothyroidism, there's no doubt that a lack of adequate thyroid hormone renders the metabolism underactive, too. Simply put, if you don't have enough fuel to run the car, you won't go anywhere. Of course, unless your thyroid is completely burned out or has been surgically removed, you might still be making some thyroid hormone and, thus, putting some fuel in your tank. But unless your T_4 and T_3 levels are normal for you, you won't have enough thyroid hormone to make all the systems in your body, including your metabolism and digestive systems, work at their optimal levels.

When your metabolism is underactive, you won't be able to process all of the food you eat in order to prevent some of it from being stored as fat in your body. This can cause weight gain. If your digestive system is slow, and you experience constipation and bloating, along with an uncomfortable feeling that everything is "backed up" inside of you, you might also gain more weight.

Body Mass Index Table

Height (Inches)	Normal						Overweight					Obese										Extreme Obesity														
BMI	19	20	21	22	23	24	25	26	27	28	29	30	31	32	33	34	35	36	37	38	39	40	41	42	43	44	45	46	47	48	49	50	51	52	53	54
												Body Weight (pounds)																								
58	91	96	100	105	110	115	119	124	129	134	138	143	148	153	158	162	167	172	177	181	186	191	196	201	205	210	215	220	224	229	234	239	244	248	253	258
59	94	99	104	109	114	119	124	128	133	138	143	148	153	158	163	168	173	178	183	188	193	198	203	208	212	217	222	227	232	237	242	247	252	257	262	267
60	97	102	107	112	118	123	128	133	138	143	148	153	158	163	168	174	179	184	189	194	199	204	209	215	220	225	230	235	240	245	250	255	261	266	271	276
61	100	106	111	116	122	127	132	137	143	148	153	158	164	169	174	180	185	190	195	201	206	211	217	222	227	232	238	243	248	254	259	264	269	275	280	285
62	104	109	115	120	126	131	136	142	147	153	158	164	169	175	180	186	191	196	202	207	213	218	224	229	235	240	246	251	256	262	267	273	278	284	289	295
63	107	113	118	124	130	135	141	146	152	158	163	169	175	180	186	191	197	203	208	214	220	225	231	237	242	248	254	259	265	270	278	282	287	293	299	304
64	110	116	122	128	134	140	145	151	157	163	169	174	180	186	192	197	204	209	215	221	227	232	238	244	250	256	262	267	273	279	285	291	296	302	308	314
65	114	120	126	132	138	144	150	156	162	168	174	180	186	192	198	204	210	216	222	228	234	240	246	252	258	264	270	276	282	288	294	300	306	312	318	324
66	118	124	130	136	142	148	155	161	167	173	179	186	192	198	204	210	216	223	229	235	241	247	253	260	266	272	278	284	291	297	303	309	315	322	328	334
67	121	127	134	140	146	153	159	166	172	178	185	191	198	204	211	217	223	230	236	242	249	255	261	268	274	280	287	293	299	306	312	319	325	331	338	344
68	125	131	138	144	151	158	164	171	177	184	190	197	203	210	216	223	230	236	243	249	256	262	269	276	282	289	295	302	308	315	322	328	335	341	348	354
69	128	135	142	149	155	162	169	176	182	189	196	203	209	216	223	230	236	243	250	257	263	270	277	284	291	297	304	311	318	324	331	338	345	351	358	365
70	132	139	146	153	160	167	174	181	188	195	202	209	216	222	229	236	243	250	257	264	271	278	285	292	299	306	313	320	327	334	341	348	355	362	369	376
71	136	143	150	157	165	172	179	186	193	200	208	215	222	229	236	243	250	257	265	272	279	286	293	301	308	315	322	329	338	343	351	358	365	372	379	386
72	140	147	154	162	169	177	184	191	199	206	213	221	228	235	242	250	258	265	272	279	287	294	302	309	316	324	331	338	346	353	361	368	375	383	390	397
73	144	151	159	166	174	182	189	197	204	212	219	227	235	242	250	257	265	272	280	288	295	302	310	318	325	333	340	348	355	363	371	378	386	393	401	408
74	148	155	163	171	179	186	194	202	210	218	225	233	241	249	256	264	272	280	287	295	303	311	319	326	334	342	350	358	365	373	381	389	396	404	412	420
75	152	160	168	176	184	192	200	208	216	224	232	240	248	256	264	272	279	287	295	303	311	319	327	335	343	351	359	367	375	383	391	399	407	415	423	431
76	156	164	172	180	189	197	205	213	221	230	238	246	254	263	271	279	287	295	304	312	320	328	336	344	353	361	369	377	385	394	402	410	418	426	435	443

Courtesy of the National Heart, Lung, and Blood Institute Information Center

Thankfully, once you are on an adequate level of thyroid hormone (T_4 alone, or a combination of T_4 and T_3), you should find it easier to digest and metabolize what you eat, and it will become easier to manage your weight. The pounds that you gained before and during your initial supplemental hormone treatment should eventually come off, as long as you maintain a healthful diet and exercise appropriately. If, however, you find that it is very difficult to lose those extra pounds, further investigation into the cause for them and steps beyond the thyroid medication you are taking might be called for.

More reasons for weight gain

There are other hypothyroid-related reasons why you might gain more than the "average" five to ten pounds from lacking adequate thyroid hormone. Oftentimes, these are not as easily treated as the weight gain directly attributed to low thyroid hormone levels because they are more closely linked with your eating habits, emotional and psychological state, upbringing and genetic factors, and other lifestyle issues. For example, if your hypothyroid-induced fatigue is overwhelming, you might be so tired that you stop exercising. This lack of movement can cause muscle atrophy and, with your slower metabolism, you might gain much more weight than if you were even moderately active. Exercising can become so uncomfortable or distasteful that you might stop altogether, further exacerbating your body's weakness.

Depression can trigger eating disorders, or you might rely on fast foods for convenience's sake because you don't have the desire (or the energy) to cook for yourself. The food you eat is your fuel, so if you ingest fatty, salty, sugary foods, your body will probably process a lot of it as fat, and, again, you will gain weight that is not easily taken off.

Other unhealthful cycles can lead to weight gain, too. If you eat for reasons other than genuine hunger (for example, if your response to stress is to eat—and living with a chronic illness certainly brings on a lot of stress) you must carefully monitor your diet, or you could gain a lot of extra pounds. Unhappiness over your body image can trigger a feeling of helplessness and lead to bingeing just to make yourself "feel better" (which, in reality, it does not). Weight gain around certain times of the year is common, too, especially during the holiday-season "crunch time." And if you work in a job where business meals are common, you might know how tempting it is to eat plentifully if your employer or someone else is treating you!

Another factor that might influence your propensity to gain weight is the way you were brought up (what foods your family consumed), as well as whether obesity "runs in" your family. There are medical studies going on now to pinpoint the genetic components to weight gain and the difficulty in taking off the pounds.[1] There are even drug studies being conducted to see if there can be some medication that can deter the effects of genetics on a person's inability to get to and maintain a normal, healthy weight. But these might take time to develop; in the meantime, you still need to take steps to do the best you can to take care of yourself and your health. If there is a strong genetic link in your family to weight gain, you might have a difficult time rising above it. Eating habits that are ingrained in us from childhood will also be difficult to break. But as with all healthful cycles, with honesty, perseverance, and discipline, you can get hold of your particular weight issues and turn them around.

Anorexia nervosa and bulimia nervosa

Hypothyroid patients are not immune to developing eating disorders. The two most common are anorexia nervosa and bulimia nervosa. In anorexia nervosa, a person might fast frequently, be picky about the food he or she eats, and engage in excessive exercise. In bulimia nervosa, a person binges and then purges the food from his or her stomach by inducing vomiting and/or taking laxatives. In some cases, a person might go from anorexic activity to bulimic and back again.

Both anorexia and bulimia are serious conditions and can have severe effects upon your health and life, sometimes causing death. If you think you might be anorexic or bulimic, please seek competent medical help right away. Talk to your doctor, or a trusted counselor, or an organization such as the National Eating Disorders Association (www.nationaleatingdisorders. org). There is no shame in developing one of these eating disorders, and caring, compassionate help is available for you, if you ask for it.

Controlling weight gain

"Being hypothyroid doesn't mean that you can't lose weight," says Elliot G. Levy, M.D. "It just means that you will have to work harder at it."

Honesty is the biggest factor in being able to analyze your weight and fitness situation and find ways to cope with it better. Using the BMI chart and discussing where you fall into it with your doctor and where you should be is a good way to start taking the problem out of your hands and collaborating with a trained medical professional. Ask to be given a stress test to see where you stack up to people in the same age and weight/height ranges. Work with a psychologist or counselor to discover the emotional bases for your eating habits and develop a game plan to eat more healthfully.

Once you and your medical team have determined how much weight you need to lose and how you are going to lose it, establish your responsibility and role in your overall weight-loss program. Acknowledge that, although you don't have control over becoming hypothyroid, you do have control over what food you eat and when you eat it. Of course, there are many emotional, psychological, and even socioeconomic reasons for overeating, or having a less-than-nutritious diet. But if you carefully analyze these things, you can see them clearly and learn to manage them so that they benefit you rather than bring you down.

Before the thyroid replacement hormone kicks in fully is an excellent time to use your health journal to chart when you eat, why you eat, and what you eat. Note the times that you overate, ate something that wasn't nutritious, or ate because of reasons other than hunger. Later, when you see how much weight you lose from bringing your thyroid levels back into the normal range, you can analyze your "eating log" and determine where you need to make changes so that you can reach a healthy weight and embrace good eating habits. Just as there are unhealthy cycles, there are also healthy ones. You can identify what is best for you and then take steps to do that, especially where your diet is concerned. And you will reap the health benefits for the rest of your life.

When you have an idea of your eating patterns and the emotions connected with it, you can begin to explore the myriad of weight-loss programs, books, and organizations available today. Your budget will also have an impact on what weight-loss road you take. Some residential programs completely overhaul your body and emotional response to food, but they can be exorbitantly pricey. Likewise, weight-loss programs where you have to buy specific brands of food can also be extremely expensive, and many people regain their lost pounds when they stop participating in them.

Dieting requires a lot of willpower, and many people find that if they have a "buddy," or counselor, they are more successful at it. Weight Watchers encourages attendance at meetings and regular "weigh-ins." Overeaters Anonymous also has meetings and many people find them helpful. Your doctor might have other ideas, too, and you should discuss your weight worries with him or her all along the way, being aware that your overeating or improper diet might be connected to many things other than hypothyroidism.

"A lot of people who are overweight eat not because they are hungry, but because they're tired, happy, bored, sad . . ." says Dr. Levy. "Until you learn other strategies to deal with these things, you won't be able to lose the weight completely and keep it off."

Supplements, "miracle treatments," and you

There are many weight-loss supplements, gizmos, and gadgets on the market today. Many advertisements show remarkable "before" and "after" photos, and testimonials sound fantastic. But do they really work?

Recently, the Federal Trade Commission, together with the Food and Drug Administration, issued a warning to consumers about so-called "miracle" weight-loss products.[2] Many of them don't begin to live up to their claims. And although they profess spectacular results, in many cases once people stop taking the supplements or doing the exercises, they end up regaining the weight they lost. Some supplements are extremely expensive, others are very uncomfortable, and a few are dangerous. Sometimes, too, certain substances can cause serious side effects. Ephedra, for example, has been linked to heart arrhythmia, heart attack, and death. For a hypothyroid patient, whose metabolism is already dysfunctional, taking a supplement that "speeds you up" can interfere with your thyroid treatment, tax your internal organs, and potentially lead to serious health side effects.

Before you invest in weight-loss supplements, make sure that you have a complete list of all the ingredients and the amounts of those ingredients and show it to your doctor. Get his or her okay before you begin taking anything, and make sure that you communicate with your physician on a regular basis if you do decide to take the supplements. *Do not* take additional thyroid hormone medication to lose weight. Only take the dosage that your doctor feels is necessary to keep your thyroid levels in the normal range.

Operation Cure-All

A GOOD source of solid information regarding the truth in the many health claims made on the Internet is the Federal Trade Commission's Operation Cure-All. Here, the FTC, in cooperation with other governmental agencies, provides consumers with facts about these claims, and gives consumers a way to complain if they have experienced side effects or other problems with over-the-counter "health" supplements. You can find Operation Cure-All at www.ftc.gov.

Coping with weight loss

In some cases, if the reason for weight gain is deeply rooted in personal trauma, weight *loss* can be as difficult to cope with as obesity.

"Some women who are very overweight have had real issues of abuse and/or rejection by a parent," says Dr. Levy. "This is a theme that is prevalent among very young women, but it's hard to talk about. They might repress it and it won't enter their minds, but it affects them. A person will be in an intensive program, lose weight, and then realize they were hiding behind their shield of obesity when someone finds them attractive. They won't know how to deal with it."

If this is true for you, it is vitally important that you realize you must do what is most healthful for yourself. You *deserve* to be taken care of. A good doctor who is compassionate will listen to your concerns and guide you to seek proper help in order to come to terms with the trauma within you so that you can cope with it and truly take good care of yourself.

IN A SENTENCE:

> *Weight gain due in part or directly to hypothyroidism can be dealt with by being vigilant, honest with yourself, seeking help where you need it, and by being patient with your body as it adjusts to your medical and physical treatments.*

learning

Diet and Exercise

IS THERE an ideal diet for the hypothyroid patient? And is there any way that diet can reverse hypothyroidism and "revive" the thyroid gland?

The most common cause of hypothyroidism is an auto-immune condition (Hashimoto's thyroiditis), where antibodies attack the thyroid gland and eventually "burn it out." Most doctors agree that there is no direct cause-and-effect relationship between diet and hypothyroidism. Still, this does not mean that you should eat whatever you want, disregarding proper nutrition. It is vitally important that you take care of your body inside and out, including what you eat, and that you make sure that you get all the nutrients your body needs to maintain balance and health.

The cholesterol connection

Cholesterol is a fat (lipid) that your body's cells need to function and that makes up part of your cells' membranes. It also assists in the formation of some hormones. Cholesterol is carried through your blood by proteins called **apoproteins**. Apoproteins carrying lipids are called **lipoproteins**. You have probably heard cholesterol spoken of in two ways: **low-density lipoprotein** (LDL) and **high-density lipoprotein** (HDL).

HDL is sometimes called the "good" cholesterol because it helps remove excess cholesterol from your body, preventing plaque from building up in your arteries. LDL causes fats to adhere to your arteries, and is often called the "bad" cholesterol. Ideally, you should maintain a low level of LDL cholesterol and a high level of HDL cholesterol. Many factors influence just how you go about doing this.

Because hypothyroidism can bring on **hyperocholesterolemia** (high cholesterol), you have to be especially careful to avoid foods that contain cholesterol and other fats that tend to raise it. Unsaturated fats (monounsaturated and polyunsaturated) do not usually raise blood cholesterol when eaten in moderation (however they do contain calories, which can contribute to weight gain). These are found in olive, canola, sunflower, soybean, corn, cottonseed, and peanut oils, as well as some kinds of nuts.

Saturated fats, dietary cholesterol, and trans-fatty acids all contribute to elevating LDL cholesterol. Products that contain one or more of these fats are dairy products, meats (high fat, liver and organ meats), poultry skin and fat, lard, coconut oil, egg yolks, and partially hydrogenated vegetable oil (which is often found in processed foods, bakery items, and fried foods).

Dietary Guidelines published by the U.S. government suggest that you should limit your intake of saturated fat to less than 10 percent of your total calories per day, and a total fat intake of no more than 30 percent of calories.[3] This means that a person consuming 2,000 total calories a day should take in 20 or fewer grams of saturated fat, and 65 or fewer grams of total fat.

To make sure that your cholesterol is under control, ask your doctor to check it regularly during the first year of your treatment. If it is high, develop a game plan to bring your numbers into a lower range. You might need to take cholesterol-lowering medication, or you might need to alter your diet. Getting into healthful eating habits can go a long way toward controlling your cholesterol and, thus, avoiding complications due to high LDL.

A *healthful diet*

There is a lot of press today about the dangerous effects of too much fat, salt, and sugar in the American diet and how these substances affect the overall health of the population. These cautionary stories apply to the hypothyroid person, too, and even more so to the person whose thyroid hormone is still in the process of being regulated. An underactive metabolism will have a harder time processing fat, salt, and sugar, and will store more of it in the form of fat in your body, so you need to be especially vigilant about what you eat in the early days of your thyroid hormone treatment. Also, you want to avoid the other unhealthful side effects of these substances. Too much fat can cause high cholesterol, weight gain, and related problems including coronary artery disease and peripheral vascular disease. Too much salt can cause high blood pressure and hypertension, and too much sugar can encourage tooth decay and gum disease.

How much is "too" much?

○ **Fat.** Dietary guidelines on fat recommend that we should aim for a total daily fat intake of no more than 30 percent of calories. Our total daily intake of saturated fat should be no more than 10 percent of our total daily calorie intake.

○ **Salt.** Salt is a mineral that contains sodium, a substance that, if eaten in great amounts, can raise blood pressure. Most people only need about ¼ of a teaspoon of salt per day to maintain appropriate levels in their bodies. The recommended maximum daily value of sodium is 2,400 milligrams, which is about the equivalent of 1 teaspoon of salt. In the U.S., we usually get enough sodium from everyday eating, and it is usually not necessary to add additional salt to the foods we eat.

○ **Sugars.** Sugars supply us with energy and are derived during digestion from carbohydrates. For this reason, they are an essential component of our diets. You might be surprised to know that sugars and starches occur naturally in many foods, including milk, fruit, some vegetables, and grain-containing products such as bread and cereals. Usually, the amount of sugar you eat in these products is enough for you to function adequately. Also, you benefit from the mineral and vitamin content that these foods contain. Adding extra sugar to your diet in the form of refined sugar, syrup, high-fructose corn syrup, dextrose, lactose, molasses, or honey can lead you to develop tooth decay, gain weight, and crowd from your diet other more healthful foods that your body really needs.

A truly healthful diet includes many fresh fruits and vegetables, some protein, and moderate amounts of fat (the "good" kind). It is varied enough so that you don't get bored and turn to unhealthful "snacks." It is also practical;

you should be able to eat well each day and not feel strained about sticking to something that is completely unmanageable.

Some practical diet tips

Here are some things that I've found helpful to keep my eating on track:

○ **Read labels.** In the U.S., many processed foods contain high levels of sodium, fat, and added sugar. Even so-called "healthy" frozen dinners, canned soups, and prepackaged meals can be surprisingly high in non-nutritious substances. Reviewing the labels of foods you normally eat will help you avoid too much of a bad thing and add more healthful substitutes to your diet.

○ **Write down the diet.** By keeping a food log, you will be able to track the items in your diet that contain processed or otherwise unhealthful additives. You will also see the beneficial things that you eat—fresh fruits, vegetables, lean meats and fish—and determine where you could make some healthful changes. For example, if you drink milk, you might switch to non-fat or low-fat (1percent) instead of whole milk. Likewise, low-fat cheese can be just as delicious, but not as fat-filled, as regular cheese.

○ **Plan ahead.** Don't go to the supermarket hungry or you will be more tempted to buy things you don't really want (or need). Make a list and stick to it, reviewing it for fresh, healthful foods.

○ **Cook ahead.** If you have horrible fatigue, you might opt for carry-out instead of cooking meals, especially if you have a family to feed. Prepare for this by fixing large portions of sauces (with lots of veggies) and other treats and freeze them so you always have some on hand.

○ **Embrace variety.** Varying your diet will keep you from getting bored with healthful eating. I like to take advantage of the fruits that are in season (cherry season is my favorite), so that I don't lose my taste for any one fruit. I also grow strawberries and sometimes vegetables on my balcony, which keeps fresh produce close at hand.

○ **Try new tastes.** Investigate alternative ways of seasoning food so that it isn't so bland that you don't want to eat it. There are many prepared spice blends, for example, that don't contain salt but do have great flavor. Fresh ginger can be a substitute for salt, too, and garlic and onions can add extra taste to most dishes.

○ **Work with a health professional.** In many cases, it is difficult to make changes to your diet all by yourself. Working with your doctor and a trained nutritionist can help guide you around foods that you might have trouble digesting or to which you might be allergic. They can also give you enough structure to make it through the transition from the way you have been eating to the way you should be eating.

Iodine and iodide

Iodine is an element found in much of our food, especially "iodized" salt, and is an essential component to producing thyroid hormone. In fact, about 80 percent of the body's iodine is stored in the thyroid gland and used to make T_4 and approximately 20 percent of the body's T_3.

Iodide is a component of iodine and is actively involved in signaling the thyroid gland to produce its hormones. Too little iodide will inhibit production of T_4. Too much will deter the conversion process of T_4 to T_3.

Hypothyroidism due to iodine deficiency can be commonplace in countries where diets do not contain much iodine. In the U.S., people generally consume enough iodine, so hypothyroidism due to iodine deficiency is usually not an issue. The most common cause of hypothyroidism in the U.S. and other developed countries is autoimmune in nature (Hashimoto's thyroiditis).

Nevertheless, periodically, you will hear of a "cure" for hypothyroidism that involves taking extra iodine. Unless your doctor has determined that you have an iodine deficiency, it is not a good idea to take supplements containing iodine in addition to your normal diet because too much iodine, like too little, can bring on hypothyroidism. Eating iodine-rich foods in moderation (sushi, for example) should not be a problem.

Goitrogens

One substance that is found in food and that interferes with the thyroid's ability to produce hormone is called a **goitrogen**. Goitrogens also promote development of **goiter**, the enlargement of the thyroid gland.

Some foods that contain goitrogens are cabbage, rutabaga, and green leafy vegetables. Although some sources say that goitrogens should be completely avoided, most doctors do not feel that this is necessary.

"I've never seen a patient come in with hypothyroidism because they've eaten too much cabbage," says Dr. Levy. "It really has to do more with certain areas of the world where they are borderline iodine deficient to begin with. In the U.S., it is an overstated situation."

In fact, avoiding goitrogen-containing foods can deprive your diet of much-needed nutrients and variety. Again, unless your doctor advises you to avoid certain foods, or you have allergies or don't like a particular food, you should try to balance your diet and consume fruits, vegetables, fats, and proteins that will help you maintain a healthy weight and balance.

Exercise

A good weight-loss or maintenance program includes a healthful diet *and* some form of exercise with an aerobic component. However if you are very fatigued from the trauma of reaching your diagnosis, as well as from hypothyroidism itself, you might not feel like exercising much. That's understandable, and there's a physiological reason for it, as well as a psychological reason. Because your metabolism is slower, and your muscles aren't getting the thyroid hormone that they should to function adequately, your whole body is running on less fuel than it needs. You might also get a lot of muscle cramps, particularly in your calves, which is also a by-product of hypothyroidism and quite painful. Psychologically, you might be depressed or don't want to exercise for fear of hurting yourself. This, too, is understandable; we're sick enough without wanting to do something that's distasteful or that we fear might hurt us further.

Still, there are many good reasons why exercise is beneficial to you now and in the long run. If you were hyperthyroid before becoming hypothyroid, you know that your overactive thyroid gland might have made you predisposed to developing osteoporosis. Exercise can help combat bone deterioration due to osteoporosis.

A strong cardiovascular system is important for preventing heart disease, and exercise is a vital component in an overall healthful heart plan. It is also good for your lungs, your muscle strength, your range of motion, and your sense of well-being and positive body image.

But where do you begin?

An exercise plan

Before you begin any exercise routine, you should discuss what you want to do with your doctor. Some tips for getting started are:

○ **Talk with your doctor.** If you are severely hypothyroid, you might have to restrict your physical activities because of the strain exercise could put on your heart and lungs. Ask your doctor what kind of exercise you can engage in and stick to that program until your thyroid hormone is under better control.

○ **Go slowly.** Find a physical therapist or exercise professional who can show you some simple, easy stretches to keep your range of motion normal, even if you don't feel like exercising more strenuously. Do these at least once a day, perhaps folding them into your meditation and/or prayer routine. Also, the Arthritis Foundation (www.arthritis.org) has a wonderful low-impact exercise program called **P**eople with **A**rthritis **C**an **E**xercise (PACE). Even if you don't have arthritis, you could benefit from their approach to movement and protecting sensitive parts of your body.

○ **"No pain, no strain."** Exercise shouldn't be painful, nor should it leave you feeling worse than when you started. It should help you maintain muscle tone and invigorate you. If you feel pain while exercising, stop and talk with your doctor before proceeding.

○ **Think of your whole life as an athletic endeavor.** Bring exercise into your daily life by parking farther from your destination and walking into the store or taking the stairs up to work. Learn how to lift and carry heavy objects properly (ask a physical therapist or exercise professional) so that you don't strain yourself, but instead give your muscles a bit of a workout.

For those who don't like to exercise

Okay, I'll confess. I was the kind of high school student who'd do almost *anything* not have to take gym class. For me, exercise wasn't something I *liked* to do. And when I reached adulthood, well, I just did not feel comfortable exercising in a private (or public) gym surrounded by people who always seemed *way* fitter than I was.

Now, however, I have realized that the benefits from exercising outweigh the negatives. Here are some ways I've found to make exercise work for me:

○ **Make exercise fun**. I don't like running on a treadmill or riding a stationary bike, so I walk or workout with exercise tapes set to fun and energizing music. Dancing is another good way to get a great cardiovascular workout and have a good time, too.

○ **Make it a game.** Playing tennis with friends is a great way to socialize *and* get a good workout. So is golfing, bowling, pickup basketball, and even table tennis (Ping-Pong).

○ **Vary the routine**. Exercise becomes a chore when it's done the same way each time. Varying the rhythm of it, or the place and time, helps make it different—and fun.

○ **Don't worry about the image**. Okay, I know I'll never fit into the skin-tight leotard and big hair image of the "perfect" exerciser. But you know what? After losing half my eyebrows to hypothyroidism and my hair to lupus, and after putting on those "pesky" five to ten extra pounds of thyroid weight, well, I don't *care* about how my image stacks up to the "gym divas"! All I care about is doing what's best for my body. And if the "best" is to exercise, well then, I'll find a way to do it!

○ **Make it simple and inexpensive.** Before you invest in expensive equipment or a pricey spa membership, give your exercise routine a trial run (some spas will even allow this). Be realistic about how much you will use your membership and/or whether you will be diligent about working out on the piece of equipment that's taking up your living room. I have opted for a simple (videos at home or a walk around town) option and probably get a better benefit from it than if I'd spent hundreds of dollars.

IN A SENTENCE:

> *A good diet and adequate exercise are vitally important for everyone, but especially for the person who is hypothyroid.*

FIRST-WEEK MILESTONE

By the end of the first week, you have already met one of the greatest challenges facing you as a hypothyroid patient: learning the basics about your condition.

○ YOU'VE LEARNED ABOUT WHAT HYPO-THYROIDISM IS AND THE CONNECTION BETWEEN YOUR LOW THYROID HORMONE PRODUCTION AND YOUR METABOLISM.

○ YOU'VE LEARNED THAT BEING HYPO-THYROID IS NOT YOUR FAULT AND NEITHER YOU NOR YOUR FAMILY MEMBERS SHOULD FEEL GUILTY BECAUSE YOU ARE ILL.

○ YOU KNOW THAT THERE ARE MILLIONS OF PEOPLE THROUGHOUT THE U.S. AND THE WORLD WHO ARE ALSO HYPOTHYROID, AND YOU KNOW YOU ARE NOT ALONE.

○ YOU'VE LEARNED ABOUT THE DIFFERENT KINDS OF SUPPLEMENTAL THYROID HOR-MONE AND ARE CONFIDENT YOU CAN UNDERSTAND THEM WHEN YOU SPEAK WITH YOUR DOCTOR.

○ YOU UNDERSTAND THAT, ALTHOUGH YOU DO NOT FEEL WELL, THERE ARE MANY THINGS THAT YOU CAN DO AND MANY THINGS THAT YOU CAN CONTROL TO MAKE YOUR LIFE BETTER.

Tired of Being Tired

ONE OF the most frustrating things about the fatigue that comes from hypothyroidism is that everyone you talk to says *they* are tired, too, as if what you're feeling isn't unusual. But if you have been living with hypothyroid fatigue, you know that it is very different from "regular" fatigue, and much more difficult to cope with.

"I know by watching the people in my house, I can definitely say my fatigue is not normal," says Pamela G. "You can feel it in your bones."

"Before I started my supplemental thyroid hormone treatment, when I'd get tired, I'd reach for that backup energy, but most of the time it wouldn't kick in," says Joe B. "I remember thinking, 'Is this what getting old is all about?'"

No rest for the weary

That persistent, numbing feeling when you don't think you can keep your eyes open can be a powerful signal that your thyroid gland is not functioning properly. But it doesn't necessarily lead to a good night's sleep and a feeling of refreshment in the morning. That makes it even more aggravating when people counter your talk about being tired with, "Oh, I'm tired, too. Go to bed early, like I do, and you'll feel better."

Hearing people express their fatigue in those terms might make you angry, because you know that your feeling of being exhausted is different from theirs. The kind of overwhelming, muscle-numbing exhaustion that is with you all the time is not going to go away with a nap once a week. It is not going to go away if you spend twelve hours in bed each night. It is not going to go away until your thyroid hormone is in balance and you have addressed other health issues that have cropped up partly or wholly because of it.

Another thing that can make you angry about being tired all the time is your inability to keep up with activities that would make you a lot happier. Parties, weddings, even a simple game of softball in the evening after work— all of these and more seem impossible because you are just too tired to summon up the energy to do them. The effects of this can also be further worrisome. Friends might stop inviting you to do things because they think you don't want to be with them. You might start losing more muscle tone because you aren't getting enough exercise. Your depression can get worse, and your feeling of isolation can be crushingly horrible. Worst of all, you might be caught in a vicious cycle: You are tired of being tired so you get more tired.

Pace yourself

A valuable lesson to learn early on in your recovery from the acute symptoms of hypothyroidism is to find ways to pace yourself so that you don't have to cut out all of the activities that you enjoy. The best way to begin to do this is to write down all the activities you do in a day. You'll be surprised at how exhausting doing *that* can be, and you'll probably marvel at how packed your schedule is.

Once you've written down a week's worth of activities, cross off those things that could be put off until you have more time, or things that are unnecessary and sap your precious energy. For example, maybe you don't have to do laundry twice a week; if you purchase a few extra towels, perhaps you could get by with doing it once a week. Prepare enough food at one time so that you can freeze some of it and only have to heat it up on the days when you're too tired to cook.

If you see that you're spending a lot of time on the phone, decide to let your answering machine take your calls during a part of the day and return those calls when you have enough energy. This will help you weed out the telemarketers and other unwanted calls, but still keep in touch with friends and loved ones.

Find ways to pace your favorite activities so that you can still do them, or substitute other activities for them so you can get the same benefit without overtaxing yourself. Perhaps you cannot play tennis three times a week, but you can play once if you rest enough on the days leading up to and afterward. Or if aerobic exercise is beyond your capability right now, ask your friends if they will go for a walk with you instead. Use that time to stretch your legs and maintain your emotional contact with people who are dear to you.

Determine when your best waking hours are and schedule the most important things you need to do during that time. Try not to do anything that requires a lot of attention when you are at your most tired.

Learn to say "no"

If you are a parent, you work outside the home, or you volunteer a lot, you might have difficulty saying no. But now that you are hypothyroid, you will need to change the way you react to requests for help. You will need to protect your energy so that you can be effective at things that are most important to you and your loved ones.

There are many different ways to say no so that you don't burn bridges. Here are a few:

○ **Offer a compromise.** If you can't do something, offer an alternative. Volunteer for the afternoon carpool instead of the early morning one. Send out a mailing for your favorite charity instead of being on hand at a lengthy, energy-zapping event.

○ **Be honest about your condition.** You don't have to "be brave": Explain that you have an illness that causes severe fatigue and ask for understanding until you get your hypothyroidism under control.

○ **Express your regret.** Follow up your "I can't" with "I'm sorry, I'd like to." Let your friends and family know that you're not just avoiding them, and keep your relationships emotionally close.

Prioritize

When you have a chronic illness, you have to learn to be very firm in what is *essential* for you to do, what is *important,* and what is *optional.*

Essential things include tasks that make your life healthful, safe, and financially and emotionally stable. Examples are:

○ Taking care of your health
○ Taking care of your family
○ Paying your bills
○ Maintaining your relationships
○ Performing well on the job (if you are working) and finding some way to be productive even if you're not working.

Important things include activities that you already enjoy, such as:
○ Hobbies and sports that you share with friends and family
○ Volunteer activities, especially if you have a position of responsibility

Optional activities include:
○ Joining a new organization
○ Taking up a new hobby
○ Taking on added responsibility unnecessarily at work

Throughout each day, you will be faced with making decisions about activities that are essential, important, or optional for you. Remember that you can't do everything (not even healthy people can do that). You need to decide among all your choices how and where you will spend your precious energy. Like never before, you have to manage your time, indeed your whole life.

Sleeping

Unfortunately, a "good night's sleep" doesn't often bring the refreshment for us that it does for healthier people. There are ways we can improve our sleep time, however, so that we do get the most possible from it.

○ Make your sleeping room restful. Minimize the distractions (television, computer, radio, books) in your bedroom so that you can truly focus on falling asleep. Also, your bedroom (or sleep room) should be quiet and dark and comfortable (neither too hot nor too cold).

○ Set aside true sleep time. "Catching a few zzz's" doesn't often bring as much rest as setting aside a block of time when you can relax and not feel as though you are being jarred awake.

○ Prepare for sleep time. Have a routine that is both restful and focused before you go to bed. Take a bubble bath, do some yoga or stretches, listen to soothing music, let your husband or wife massage your back, or just visualize a full, refreshing night's sleep.

○ Let the answering machine take messages.

○ Wake up to soothing music or just sleep-lazy stretching so that you can gradually rejoin the day.

Be patient

As your medication begins to work, the sharpness of your fatigue should lessen. You will also be more productive during your "up" times. Expect ups and downs, as your doctor works at adjusting your medication and your thyroid hormone levels adjust, too. Be patient, but positive—you *will* feel better!

IN A SENTENCE:

> Hypothyroid fatigue is very difficult to cope with so it is important for you to take care of yourself, set boundaries, learn to say "no" and prioritize the activities on which you spend your energy each day.

learning

Physical Improvements

WEIGHT GAIN, hair loss, lackluster skin, loss of muscle tone—these are some of the unattractive affects of hypothyroidism that you can see when you look in the mirror. And there's nothing like feeling unattractive to assail your emotional and spiritual health, too. When you think you look bad, you *feel* bad. And when you feel bad, you are less likely to take extra steps to make the most of your appearance, in spite of your illness. Now that you've learned what's happening inside your body, you can take positive steps to improve the outside effects of hypothyroidism.

The hairy truth for women

Although it is not easy to let go of our hair, because of hypothyroidism, we might not have any choice. If the creams and injections don't work, we have to be proactive and find ways to improve our appearance in spite of balding and losing half of our eyebrows.

There are many attractive wigs on the market now, and they vary enough in price to make them affordable to most budgets. It is not necessary to get a natural hair wig. In fact, these can be more difficult to take care of than synthetic wigs.

If you lose so much hair that you need to get a wig, here are some suggestions for finding the perfect coiffure:

○ Make your shopping expedition into something fun. Take along a good friend and get her to try on some wigs, too. Sharing in the experience can be an enjoyable way to make it less emotionally painful.

○ Consider changing your hair color, style, or length. It is extremely easy to do this using wigs because you don't have to mess with curlers, hair dyes, or expensive trips to the beauty salon. You can also have the wig you own trimmed or restyled if you want to have a change.

○ Invest in a good wig brush (it has metal bristles instead of boar or nylon) and ask about how to care for your wig at home. Usually this is as easy as washing it out with your regular shampoo, but you might want to purchase some wig-specific shampoo instead.

○ If your budget will allow, purchase two wigs so that you can wear one while the other is drying. This is also a great idea if you think you'll want to change your "look" from one day to the next. You might be able to finally find out if blondes do have more fun!

The life span of a wig is usually about a year. After that time, they can look very worn (please pardon the pun). If you need to wear a wig over a long period of time, think about buying more than one and rotating them so that they will last. If you can't afford to do that, think about investing in a wig once a year and donating your old one to a homeless shelter or other nonprofit agency. You can probably take a tax deduction for the donation, and you'll be helping someone in the process.

The hairy truth for men

Men go through many of the same emotions as women when they lose their hair, however society is generally much more tolerant of balding men than of women. If you don't want to go around without some kind of hair covering, there are wonderful toupees and other hairpieces available that can provide great relief.

Unconventional sources for wigs and other hair coverings

Some cities have one or more stores devoted to hair coverings for men and women. Other sources include the American Cancer Society's "tlc" catalogue (see Resources section for the contact information), which carries wigs, falls, scarves, and hats for women who have undergone chemotherapy due to breast cancer.

Many hospitals have boutiques that carry items for men and women who have lost their hair due to alopecia and chemotherapy. Their prices are often lower than in a general retail store, and their selection is usually very attractive.

Theatrical costume shops are another great source for finding wigs and hairpieces, especially of a more "exotic" nature. These are also good places to find makeup and get tips on coping with some of the skin and other appearance issues associated with hypothyroidism.

Skin inside and out

"My skin would get so dry that you could write your name on it," says Lidia Q. "I never used to use moisturizer, but now I carry it around in my purse and reapply it during the day. That gets rid of the itch. The itchiness is annoying."

The flaky, itchy skin that often accompanies hypothyroidism can be unsightly as well as uncomfortable. Fortunately, we live in an era where there are many products available to soothe and strengthen your skin against these symptoms. Finding the right skin lotion and care regimen will take time, but it is worth it when you see the benefits to being patient and careful about what you use and how you use it.

Soap, even the "mild" variety, can be very drying, even if your skin tends to be oily. You are better off using a good skin cleanser that does not contain soap products and drying fragrances. Ask your dermatologist to recommend one, or ask your friends what they use. Visit a drug store and/or department store and ask for samples of products that you can try so you don't spend a lot of money for things that you will only use once or twice and then discard.

If you decide to purchase products you see advertised in magazines or on television, look beyond the "hype" and determine if what the advertisers say seems reasonable. I am usually very skeptical about claims that creams or lotions will "erase aging completely." Instead, I opt for a steady, nourishing kind of skin care that gives me just the moisture and cleanliness I need without all the bells and whistles.

When you clean your face, use lukewarm water (not hot), and pat your skin dry with a soft towel (don't scrub). Afterward, use a moisturizer formulated specifically for the face; body moisturizers tend to be too heavy to use on your more delicate facial skin.

Everyone should be careful about sun exposure, but if you have skin problems because of your hypothyroidism, you should be especially cautious. When you are outdoors, wear a good sunscreen because sun exposure can dry and damage your skin. Apply it once at the beginning of the day and then periodically throughout the day because some of it might rub off during the normal course of your activities.

If you are going to be outside, wear a hat and other protective clothing (don't forget about protecting the back of your neck, hands, and feet). And choose your outdoors activities so that you are out of the sun at its peak— usually between 10 A.M. and 4 P.M.

Eating properly and drinking enough water will help your skin thrive, too. The right balance of nutrition and cleansing will help you establish a "glow" that will be with you throughout your early days of treatment and beyond.

Eye care

Hyperthyroidism, specifically Graves' disease, can cause eye problems, including exophthalmos, a condition where the eyes "bulge" outward. Such troubles are rarer in people with hypothyroidism. Still, it is a good idea to get your eyes checked by an ophthalmologist to rule out any eye involvement. Also, consult with your doctor and an ophthalmologist before going ahead with any kind of laser eye surgery.

A new you!

Coping with all the physical changes that come with hypothyroidism is hard. But if you keep in mind that you can do things to improve your skin, hair, and overall appearance, you can ease some of your worries. And, who knows? You might discover a new "look" that's unique, wonderful, and completely "you"!

IN A SENTENCE:

> *Although hypothyroidism can bring some unsightly and unwanted physical changes, you can take advantage of many cosmetic options to conceal them and even improve your body and your self-image.*

Analyzing Information

IN THE first days and weeks after your diagnosis and start of treatment, you were bombarded with so much information that you barely had time to think about it all. One of the good parts of this book is that the information is broken down into manageable pieces for you—day-by-day, week-by-week. But still you might find yourself on information overload. Don't worry about this—it's perfectly normal. I still get a little lost when I navigate the Internet for too long, moving from site to site, from link to link. Indeed, it seems as though there is an ocean of information out there—and sometimes my compass needs an overhaul! Going back to the basics of information acquisition and analysis is an excellent way to take some of the confusion out of the huge body of data and advice that we come in contact with once we are diagnosed with a chronic illness.

The search for "true" information

There are several ways to find out information about hypothyroidism. These include:

○ Medical professionals, especially endocrinologists
○ Books specific to hypothyroidism and general health
○ Drug company literature, including Web sites

○ Internet searches, which include "public" information and professional medical sites
○ News reports, magazine articles
○ Anecdotal information—stories that people tell you or that you read about

Your search for information will occur in several stages:

○ The beginning. This is when you are first diagnosed and want to know *everything* about hypothyroidism. This is also the time when you might be most likely to become confused by the onslaught of information you find. This period might last several weeks, and overlaps a bit with the whole first year of living with hypothyroidism.
○ "The First Year." During the first year following your diagnosis, you are eager to seek specific information and answers to questions concerning hypothyroidism and how it relates directly to you. This is the focus of this book.
○ Years to come. After the first year, you are more comfortable with your knowledge base. Still, you continue to learn, adding to your knowledge in the form of continued reading, building your support group of others who suffer from hypothyroidism, and keeping yourself up to date on the latest in research developments.

How to sift through information

Analyzing the data, advice, and anecdotes that you find during your search for information can be daunting. Here are some tips for separating the beneficial from the not so helpful:

○ Consider the source. Look beyond what is being told to you and consider the training, the bias, and the manner in which information is being communicated. Is the person qualified to be an "expert"? Is the organization or research group dedicated to helping patients or selling a product? Are the testimonials given by credible sources, too?
○ Cross-check the information. If someone says he or she has "THE solution" to a problem or symptom, check with other credible sources

and see if the same solution holds true with them. Go to your doctor, who has a clinical perspective on what works with patients; an agency that oversees medications and treatments (such as the Food and Drug Administration) or another qualified source.

○ Be wary of "cures" and "hidden secrets." If there *were* a cure to hypothyroidism, if it could be reversed, doctors would prescribe it. There are "gray areas," such as the T_3 controversy. But there is no cure for hypothyroidism and there is no herbal substitute for thyroid hormone.

○ Examine the data. There are scientific studies and there are anecdotal studies. It is very important that you know everything about *how* data is collected in order to be able to understand just how reliable a study is for the general population. In other words, there's a huge difference between someone saying, "All my friends say [X] works for them" and someone else saying, "We studied [a large representation of the population] over [number of years] using [scientific method], and our findings were . . ."

○ Trust your instincts. We've all heard the adage, "If something sounds too good to be true, it is." Trust that instinct in yourself and apply it to the decisions you make regarding your life and health. If you feel like you're being given a con-job, you probably are.

Asking questions

As you gather information and get to know your body better, you will still have questions. The most helpful way to formulate them is to be as specific as possible. For example, instead of asking "What can I do about my pain?" ask "My back hurts [number on a scale of 1 to 10]. The pain is [sharp, throbbing, dull ache . . .]. What can I do about it?"

Ways to help you get to "basics" are:

○ Writing down your questions
○ Talking over your questions and concerns with a trusted loved one
○ Talking with other people who are hypothyroid to hear of their experiences
○ Using your meditation and/or prayer time to delve into your inner self and gain insight into your true questions

It will take time to frame your questions specifically, but it will help you and your doctor to be exacting in the treatments and medications that can help you where it hurts. Also, as you acquire helpful answers to your questions, you will increase your sense of control over your health and your life.

IN A SENTENCE:

Asking specific questions and carefully analyzing the answers you receive are vital to gaining control of your health and thriving with hypothyroidism.

learning

More about Autoimmunity

THE CONCEPT of autoimmunity and the relationship it has with your health can be confusing. When I was diagnosed with lupus, my rheumatologist made a point of explaining that lupus, the "classic" autoimmune disease, is "the opposite of cancer, the opposite of AIDS." This helped, but it took me a while to understand just how an autoimmune condition works and what it means to my overall health.

Autoimmunity—the basics

When you have an autoimmune disease, your body produces antibodies, or proteins, that attack a certain part or parts of your body. In Hashimoto's thyroiditis, for example, your body produces antibodies to the thyroid gland and over time the gland "burns itself out," or ceases to produce thyroid hormone. This reaction is very much like being allergic to part or parts of yourself; and it can be extremely damaging.

Autoimmune diseases as a category of illness have only been identified as such fairly recently. Diseases such as lupus and hypothyroidism were recognized in the nineteenth century (some even earlier), but the autoimmune process wasn't recognized until the twentieth century. Hashimoto's thyroiditis was the first autoimmune disease to be identified as such.[1] Even more recently, diagnostic tools such as blood tests have been developed to identify and isolate the antibodies causing autoimmune reactions. As a result, research into the causes of autoimmune diseases is still in the early stages, and although there are ways to bring some autoimmune diseases under control, there are few outright cures.

Researchers suspect that there are two components that go into developing an autoimmune disease, such as lupus or Hashimoto's thyroiditis: a genetic predisposition to autoimmunity and one or more environmental "triggers" that set off the process.[2] These triggers might be stress, pollutants, illness, exposure to sunlight (in the case of lupus) or a combination of these or other factors. There is no real clear-cut evidence that specific autoimmune diseases "run" in families, though there seems to be a "trend" in some families. This means that in some families, one person might have Hashimoto's thyroiditis, another will have rheumatoid arthritis, and still another might develop insulin-dependent diabetes. In another instance, two family members might carry the gene or set of genes that give them a propensity toward systemic lupus erythematosus, but one might never develop the disease, whereas the other will.

Another confusing thing about autoimmune diseases is that they frequently overlap with one another. Someone with primary Sjogren's syndrome, an autoimmune disease where antibodies attack the glands that produce the body's moisture, such as tears and saliva, might also have Hashimoto's thyroiditis. Someone with alopecia areata could also develop Addison's disease (adrenal insufficiency). This can make diagnosis and treatment difficult, and can be frustrating for doctor and patient alike.

Hashimoto's thyroiditis and other autoimmune illnesses

The incidence of autoimmune diseases is difficult to predict. It is impossible to say that if you have Hashimoto's thyroiditis you will or will not develop another autoimmune illness. There is some indication that certain autoimmune illnesses are associated with a higher than normal rate of thyroid autoimmunity. According to the *Thyroid Signpost*, a publication of the Thyroid Society for Education and Research, these include[3]:

- ○ vitiligo (patchy loss of skin coloration)
- ○ alopecia areata
- ○ rheumatoid arthritis
- ○ myasthenia gravis (episodic muscle weakness that can affect vision, speech, swallowing, and breathing)
- ○ systemic lupus erythematosus
- ○ Addison's disease (adrenal insufficiency)
- ○ Graves' eye disease
- ○ spontaneous ovarian failure
- ○ insulin-dependent diabetes
- ○ premature gray hair
- ○ pernicious anemia (inability to absorb B_{12})

Coping with multiple autoimmune diseases is not easy. Sometimes, for example, it is difficult for me to separate my "thyroid fatigue" from my "lupus fatigue." Taking many different medications, some of which have specific dosage requirements (stipulating they not be taken with other medications, or that they be taken with or without food), also complicates life.

The more illnesses you have, the more organized you have to be, and also the more flexible because one condition might "flare," that is, be more symptomatic, than another at any given time. Keeping your health journal is vital to being able to clearly communicate with your doctor. Maintaining your nurturing relationships with loved ones and keeping your prayer and/or meditation life vibrant can also be extremely helpful.

Preventing autoimmune illnesses

Although there are no preventative measures you can take that will ensure that you do not develop another autoimmune disease, you can be watchful of your own health and how well you take care of your Hashimoto's thyroiditis.

- ○ Eating well and exercising adequately will help you maintain good body strength.

○ Keeping a positive attitude toward your life and prioritizing your activities will help you reduce stress and anxiety.

○ Monitoring your symptoms and reporting new ones or exacerbation of current ones to your doctor will help you catch a potential problem early.

○ Continuing your education will give you the knowledge and awareness to recognize health issues and the latest developments in how to treat them.

IN A SENTENCE:

Having Hashimoto's thyroiditis doesn't necessarily mean you will develop another autoimmune disease, but it does mean you should be aware of the possibility and tell your doctor if you develop any new symptoms.

Work and Hypothyroidism

HOW YOU feel physically and emotionally has a tremendous impact on your ability to work. Once your body begins adjusting to your thyroid medication, you should start to see some improvement in your energy level and ability to concentrate. You will feel more productive, too, and your attitude should be more positive. But until your thyroid levels are in balance, you might need to make adjustments to the pace at which you work and to the degree to which you take on new responsibilities. If you have some flexibility at your workplace, this might be easy. If you don't have flexibility, it might be more of a challenge.

Work factors that might affect hypothyroidism

Most jobs are stressful in some way, but those jobs that are very stressful might take more of a toll on your health, especially if your hypothyroidism is severe. Jobs with long hours and a high responsibility level could tax your overfatigued metabolism. Physical work might be difficult for you if your muscle tone and weight have become compromised.

You and your doctor are the best judges of what is appropriate for you to do in your condition. Early on in your treatment for hypothyroidism, you should discuss with your doctor the work that you do and try to determine how it affects you now. Perhaps you will need to make temporary adjustments while you are getting your thyroid hormone in balance. Or perhaps the reality of having a chronic illness leads you to consider a job or career change.

Should you change jobs?

When you have a chronic illness, you begin to take stock of all aspects of your life: the state of your health, the way you live, your relationships, and your work. Many people, after much introspection, decide to change their jobs or careers to do things that have more meaning to them. They realize that life is short, health is precious, and time should be spent in pursuits that bring fulfillment to themselves and others.

Although sometimes we get mired in a way of life that makes it difficult for us to think of changing jobs, there is always a way to go from a line of work you aren't excited about to something that brings you joy. Several factors go into making up a plan of action. These include:

○ **Your skills.** What you are good at, what you need training for, what you aren't so good at. Take into account grades in school, professional achievements and awards, as well as "intangibles," such as how easily certain things come to you, how precise you can be at a job, and how you view your success with a given task or profession.

○ **Your finances.** What your budget will allow in terms of career changing, additional education/training, the needs of you and your family.

○ **Your desire**. What is it you really want to do? What is your dream job? Is there something you've been putting off doing—the career you'd like to do "someday" or "when you retire"?

○ **Your determination**. You might *want* to do something, but are you determined enough to make it a reality? Do you have the right amount of discipline and conviction? Do you have the support of your loved ones?

You are in control

Changing jobs requires planning and tenacity. Changing careers requires a lot of extra work and dedication. Only you know what is in your heart to do, and only you can be honest with yourself about your talents, desires, and financial situation. But beyond this, remember you are in control of the education you get, the contacts you make, the work you ultimately achieve. With this in mind, let your introspection be one of hope and positive forethought. Picture yourself in your ideal work situation and do something, one thing, each day to get yourself there. Each day adds up. Each thing builds upon the next. You have control of all of that.

IN A SENTENCE:

> *Having a chronic illness can make you reevaluate where you should be in work and career, and you can decide to make changes based on where you want to be and what your talents enable you to do.*

learning

Disability and the Thyroid-Friendly Workplace

YOU WILL probably not be permanently disabled due to hypothyroidism. In fact, you might never be disabled at all. However, if your symptoms are severe, you might have to take short-term leave from work so that you can allow you body a less stressful environment in which to adjust to your medication and begin to heal. Although you might not want to take time off, you might find that taking advantage of family leave, accrued vacation and sick time, and other options might help you recover more quickly and be back to a better level of functioning (and productivity) sooner.

Discussing work with your physician

The decision to take time off from work is one that ultimately you will have to make. But your doctor's input is invaluable and necessary as you go through the process to get time off or have your application for short-term disability approved. When you speak with your doctor about whether or not you should continue to work:

○ Be candid about the things you do on the job, your work environment (is it cordial, stressful, or difficult), and what, if any, repercussions there will be if you stop working (reactions of superiors, coworkers, family members) and how these will affect you.

○ Tell your doctor whether you notice any increase in your symptoms as you do your daily work (are you exposed to harmful substances, for example).

○ Invite suggestions from your doctor about things that you could do to continue to work, or ways that your employer might accommodate you on the job.

If your doctor recommends that you stop working, weigh this information against what you truly believe is your capacity to give 100 percent to your job as you try to allow your body to heal. Are you burning bridges with your coworkers because of your moodiness? Is your job too physical for your weakened body to take? Are you so depressed that you can't function at home, let alone give your all to your work?

You should take into account any financial effect that taking a break from work will bring, and weigh this against the extent of your need to take time off. Sometimes, there is more value in resting than just "dollars and cents." But sometimes the lack of a steady, adequate income can bring extra stress and aggravate health problems.

Once you have come to your conclusion, let your doctor know what you plan to do and what he or she can expect in the way of paperwork. Work with your doctor throughout your disability to make sure that your health continues to improve in the face of your changed employment status.

Options, options

The first thing you should do if you and your doctor decide you need to take time off due to illness is to review the options that your employer offers. These are usually listed in your company's employee handbook. Sometimes, employers offer paid leave of a certain duration, depending on how long an employee has been with the company. Other times, the employer will allow unpaid leave, after an employee has used up all his or her accrued vacation, sick, and discretionary time off. This leave might be protected by the Family and Medical Leave Act (FMLA).

The FMLA is a federal act designed to allow employees to take unpaid time off to care for a spouse, parent, child, or themselves should they become ill. FMLA leave can be used for doctor's appointments and treatments (such as chemotherapy, dialysis, or regular office visits). Employees are eligible to take FMLA leave if they have "worked for their employer for at least 12 months, or worked for at least 1,250 hours over the previous 12 months, and work at a location where at least 50 are employed by the employer within 75 miles" (http://www.elaws.dol.gov/fmla/wren/faq.htm).[1] Further information is available at www.elaws.dol.gov/fmla, or by contacting the U.S. Department of Labor by calling toll-free: 1-866-4-USA-DOL.

After you know what options are open to you, consult with your boss, manager, or personnel department (whichever you feel is most appropriate to speak with) and explain briefly what you need to do. You don't really need to go into detail about your medical condition, but you might have to provide a written note or form that is filled out by your doctor to verify that your request for leave is medically necessary. It is important that you are as calm and professional as possible when you speak with your employer, and you should expect your employer to be the same toward you. If you run into problems, speak with someone in a position of authority to get some resolution. If you have a problem being approved for family and medical leave and your employer is supposed to provide it for you, you might have recourse through your state's fair housing and employment department, or through the U.S. government.

Working part-time

Your medical condition might be such that you need to cut back your work hours but don't need to stop working altogether. This has certain benefits, not the least of which are financial. You will also feel productive, even while grappling with your illness, and you will have the camaraderie of your coworkers. If your employer will allow you to work part-time, this is an excellent alternative to having to stop altogether. But be careful that you don't add an hour here or there and end up back working full-time before you can physically tolerate it.

Accommodations in the workplace

If you continue to work full-time, you might consider asking for accommodation while your thyroid hormones are getting back into balance. This might include asking for a later shift so that you can sleep longer in the morning, or requesting less stressful work when you are on the job. A good employer, one who cares about his or her employees and wants to see them succeed, will listen carefully and take your suggestions for accommodation seriously.

If you are disabled but wish to continue working, you might be protected under the Americans with Disabilities Act. The ADA covers employers with 25 or more employees, as well as those with 15 to 24 employees.[2]

As it relates to the workplace, the ADA can mandate that employers need to provide "reasonable accommodation" to employees with disabilities. These might include getting you a more comfortable workstation, adjusting your hours to allow for maximum productivity during your most wakeful hours, or other modifications that will not bring an "undue hardship" on your employer's operations. Further information about the ADA is available from the Department of Justice (contact information is included in the Resources section) and on the Web at www.disability.gov.

Job hunting

If you decide to seek other employment, go about your search as if you were well. Identify your prospects, prepare your resume, practice for interviews, and network with your contacts as you normally would. You don't even have to mention your illness in an interview, unless you feel you need special accommodation in order to perform the essential duties of the job for which you are applying.

"Essential duties" are those tasks that are necessary for successful accomplishment of the job. They can be anything from working effectively with a group, team-building, typing a certain number of words per minute, or coming up with creative solutions to problems within a certain time-frame. When you consider a job, make sure that you understand what will be required of you and gauge your physical capabilities against those requirements. If you think you will need accommodation for any of them, be up-front during the application and interview process. Convey your eagerness to do the job, but let your potential employer know that you might need a little help. Usually, employers will be enthusiastic about bringing a strong candidate on board and won't balk at making a few modifications to do this. If the employer does express doubt, consider whether you want to work for him or her anyway and act accordingly.

Before you switch jobs, take into account how you will continue your health coverage from one job to the next. If your new employer requires a "waiting period" for coverage, consider going on C.O.B.R.A. (Consolidated Omnibus Budget Reconciliation Act). Under this provision, you may continue receiving coverage under your former employer's group health insurance plan by paying the premium, plus a minimal administrative fee, for up to eighteen months. If you are disabled and receive Social Security Disability benefits, you might be eligible to receive C.O.B.R.A. for an additional eleven months. Information about C.O.B.R.A. is available at www. disability.gov and www.cobrahealth.com.

Starting a new job

Even if you are healthy, a new job can be stressful. You are getting used to a new routine, workplace, and colleagues. And life outside of work doesn't just stop while you get situated.

Make full use of all your coping skills to lessen some of the stress of a new job. Avoid taking on too much too soon or letting outside activities crowd your ability to get comfortable with your new routine. Make sure you stick to your health regimen, including your medication and exercise schedule, because you will need your health to function well on the job. And by all means celebrate your new employment and the opportunities it can bring you—accomplishments and accolades don't stop because of hypothyroidism.

Setting goals, achieving dreams

Truly, there is no need to give up your career goals or your heartfelt life dreams because you are hypothyroid. You just might have to adjust the timeline for achieving them in light of your lower energy and other symptoms. If, for example, you want to complete a course of study, you might need to take a semester off or reduce your course load for the time it takes to allow your medication to work. Perhaps you won't graduate as early as you planned, but you can still get your degree or certification. Or maybe you have thought of moving into a bigger house, but your symptoms are severe. Wait until you are stronger, and you will be able to enjoy the excitement of a new home all the more.

As difficult as it might be now to imagine making significant headway with major projects or your career path, if you hold fast to what you want to do, to what is in your heart and soul to accomplish, you will be able to do it. Or, with your new perspective on yourself, your health, and your place in the world, you might gradually replace goals that become stale with new, vibrant ones that lead you on to even greater fulfillment and achievement.

IN A SENTENCE:

> *Hypothyroidism might affect your work-life, goals, and dreams temporarily, but you should be able to achieve all that you want to with time, patience, insight, knowledge, and understanding.*

FIRST-MONTH MILESTONE

A whole month has passed since you were diagnosed, and you have begun to learn a great deal about your condition, your body's reaction to it, and how you are handling your life with hypothyroidism. Among the greatest things you've accomplished are:

- ◯ YOU'VE LEARNED TO LISTEN TO YOUR BODY AND PACE YOURSELF BETTER SO THAT THE FATIGUE DOESN'T OVERWHELM YOU AS MUCH AS IT ONCE DID.

- ◯ YOU'RE MUCH MORE CONSCIOUS ABOUT SETTING PRIORITIES AT WORK AND AT HOME, AND LEAVING TIME FOR YOURSELF TO RELAX AND ENJOY "JUST BEING."

- ◯ YOU ARE AWARE OF THE EFFECT HYPO-THYROIDISM HAS ON YOUR HAIR, SKIN, AND ELSEWHERE IN AND ON YOUR BODY, AND YOU ARE TAKING STEPS TO ALLEVIATE MANY OF THE SYMPTOMS, TAKING CARE OF YOURSELF BETTER THAN YOU EVER HAVE BEFORE.

- ◯ YOU HAVE DEVELOPED A USEFUL FRAME-WORK FOR ARTICULATING YOUR QUESTIONS AND ANALYZING THE ANSWERS THAT YOU

RECEIVE FROM FAMILY, FRIENDS, MEDICAL
PROFESSIONALS, AND OTHERS.

○ YOU FEEL LIKE THE CLOUDS HAVE PARTED
A LITTLE, AND SOME SUNSHINE AND HOPE
ARE STREAMING THROUGH.

○ YOU KNOW YOU DON'T HAVE TO GIVE UP
YOUR GOALS AND YOU ARE DEVELOPING
WAYS TO MAKE THEM ACHIEVABLE.

Sticker Shock

NOW THAT you've been living with hypothyroidism for more than a month, you have seen its impact on your finances. Doctor's bills, medication, and other health-related expenses add up and can eat into your reserve funds, especially if they come up by surprise. No doubt you are beginning to worry that your financial future might have to be more restrictive because of the ongoing nature of your illness. Now is an excellent time to strategize about how you will shoulder this added financial burden and cope with your fear and stress about your economic well-being.

The need to spend

Unless scientists find a cure for your malfunctioning thyroid gland, you are going to need to monitor your condition and take medication for the rest of your life. This means you will have ongoing medical expenses. Emotionally, it's hard to realize that you can't avoid this; no one wants to live with a chronic, life-altering disease, let alone have to pay for ongoing treatment. But it's my reality, it's your reality. And one of the first positive things to do to come to terms with this is to realize: Hypothyroidism just *"is"* in the picture.

Expenses related to hypothyroidism are like those related to eating, having shelter and clothing, and operating a car (if you need one). From now on, paying for your medication and doctor bills is a necessity of life. If you don't have a healthy balance of thyroid hormone in your body, you won't be able to function well and you could cause permanent, severe damage to your overall health and well-being.

Oddly, one of the best ways to truly accept your hypothyroidism is to accept that you have ongoing medical expenses. If you see your bills for medication and doctor's visits, you can connect emotionally with what's written on the page: You have a chronic illness. Moreover, by paying for your medication and doctors, you are taking positive steps toward a better, healthier life, and this should give you a sense of control and strength.

Another benefit to having medical expenses is that you are more likely to take better care of yourself from now on so you can avoid developing other illnesses or aggravate the condition that you have. Now more than ever, you can acknowledge the gift that is good health and do everything you can to achieve and maintain it.

So, yes, there is a positive side to negative cash flow! And it helps every so often to remind yourself of that.

Fear, stress, and finances

The term "chronic illness" can conjure up all sorts of fears about financial instability and loss of whatever home equity or savings you might have built up. However, the expenses associated with treating hypothyroidism are not overpowering and are mostly predictable (another positive!). These are:

- Monthly costs for medication.
- Regular lab tests and doctor's exams.
- Variable costs for adapting to your new life (weight-loss programs, clothing when you outgrow or become too thin to wear what you have now, lost wages if you are temporarily unable to work).

Although the diagnosis might have come as a surprise, now that you know you are hypothyroid, you should be able to plan for your future expenses with some degree of certainty. And this should help alleviate much of your fear of the impact hypothyroidism will have on your finances.

Also, as your thyroid hormone levels become better regulated, you might need to go to the doctor less frequently, so some of your expenses could actually decrease.

If you live on a slender shoestring of a budget, you might not feel fear so much as stress at how you are going to find money for even the smallest of added expenses. In the Learning section for this month, you will find some practical ways to budget for medical expenses and seek assistance when and where you need it. These things, along with your positive outlook and determination to give your health all that it needs to thrive, will help you lessen the stress and reach a better feeling about your medical condition and your financial future.

IN A SENTENCE:

> *Expenses associated with treating hypothyroidism cannot be avoided, but they are usually not high and can sometimes decrease as your disease becomes better controlled.*

learning

Budgeting for a Chronic Illness

WHEN YOU budget for a chronic illness, you need to take into account two categories of expenses: the *known* and the *unknown*.

Known expenses

The money that you spend on medication, medical insurance premiums, doctor's visits, and medical tests are *known* expenses. They might go up, they might go down. But whatever the amount, they *will* be with you.

Other known expenses are those that you incur to adapt to your disease. For example, if you have gained a lot of weight, you might need new clothes. Don't throw out your old ones just yet, however, because you might lose the weight gradually and be able to fit into them again. If your weight fluctuates drastically, consider loose-fitting clothing that you can wear at different weight levels (drawstring pants, "big" shirts, unbelted dresses).

You also might need to buy things for your bedroom, or invest in one or two wigs or other cosmetic aids. Smart shopping by doing price comparisons on what you want to buy and compromising on "nonessential" things such as color or designer name can help you save money. So, too, can clipping coupons, shopping during sales times, and swapping your current possessions with those someone else has for things you need.

Depending on your budget and the extent of your need, you might spend no money on adapting, or you might spend a lot of money. But however much you spend, you can predict what something will cost at the time you need it and plan accordingly.

Thinking creatively about your spending will help you feel less stress about your finances and give you more control over them, too.

- ○ Shop for clothing at thrift stores and consignment shops (you can take your clothing there, too, and resell it).
- ○ Swap clothes with a friend who might be gaining weight while you are losing (or vice versa).
- ○ Plant a summer garden and freeze the vegetables you harvest so you don't have to buy as many during the winter.
- ○ Steer away from eating a lot of prepackaged and prepared foods that could be harmful to your health and more costly than simple home cooking.

You will undoubtedly come up with many more ideas for cost cutting as you continue through the next weeks and months. You could even enlist the help of your family in finding ways to trim expenses; make it a game and give a modest "prize" to the person who saves the most during a given period of time. And share your knowledge: It would be terrific to tell others what you've learned about budgeting. Economical ideas are never out of fashion!

Everyday dollars

After you've lived with hypothyroidism a few months, you will have a good idea of how much your known expenses will be. Just as you would plan for food, shelter, and other monthly expenses, figure these amounts into your budget. If you have your thyroid levels monitored every three months, break down the cost of this over three months and save that amount each month so that you're not hit with the whole expense at once. Add your other expenses into your budget so that you're not strapped, but you do purchase what you need.

Unknown expenses

Each of us, at some time during our walk with a chronic illness, will play the "what if?" game.

"What if I have to be hospitalized?"

"What if I can't work?"

"What if I develop another disease, more debilitating than hypothyroidism?"

"What if I'm so sick my spouse divorces me?"

There is no way to predict any of these things with any certainty, but you should protect yourself as much as possible (without living in fear). Here are some things to keep in mind:

- ○ **Insurance.** Keeping your health, life, and other insurance current will save you the stress of wondering if your medical needs are covered and your family is taken care of.
- ○ **Savings.** Putting aside something every month, even if it is a small amount (these do add up over time), will give you a cushion when extra expenses arise.
- ○ **Health.** Paying attention to preventative healthcare will help you lessen the risk of developing other or more severe illness.
- ○ **Medical team.** Maintaining good relationships with your healthcare team can hold you in good stead if you run into financial trouble (they might work out a payment plan or lower costs for you).
- ○ **Fads.** Spending money on fad diets, supplements, or "health programs," unless you have discussed them thoroughly with your doctor, can be a good way of just throwing your money away.
- ○ **Relationships.** Being realistic about the strength of your marriage or other partnerships will help you avoid surprise when or if any of them fall apart.

Financial help

If you run into financial trouble and are having a hard time meeting your medical expenses, here are some things you can do:

- ○ Contact the manufacturer of the thyroid medication you are taking and ask to be considered for their Patient Assistance Program. In some cases, drug companies will provide necessary medication free of charge. A list of manufacturers and their contacts can be found on page 232.

○ For overall financial reorganization, consider working with your community's Consumer Credit Counseling Service. For a small fee (usually no more than twenty dollars per month), they can arrange repayment plans for your debts and consolidate your payments into one monthly sum based on your financial status.

○ Ask your doctor if you can pay on installment, or otherwise pay less for the labs and services he or she gives you. If your thyroid hormone has been under good control, ask if you can come in for office visits less regularly.

Some things to avoid are:

○ Obtaining medication and medical care from unlicensed or disreputable sources.

○ Stopping your medication and thyroid hormone monitoring without the advice of your doctor.

○ Allowing symptoms or signs of other illnesses to get worse, without speaking with your doctor about them.

Taxes

A certain portion of your medical expenses might be tax deductible. Keep your receipts and canceled checks for everything you spend relating to your health and consult with an accountant when it's tax time. Even the smallest amounts add up, and you should always try to take advantage of every legal means to lessen the cost of your disease.

IN A SENTENCE:

> *A carefully prepared budget and strategies to cut the costs of your disease where you can will help you manage the financial impact of hypothyroidism and reduce your stress and worry over your money situation.*

MONTH **3**

living

Feeling Better/
Feeling Worse

BY NOW, your thyroid medication should have brought you some relief from your symptoms of fatigue and depression. If it hasn't, you should speak with your doctor about what might be preventing you from getting better. In most cases, however, by the third month of taking supplemental thyroid hormone, you should notice some progress. A quick review of your health journal will show you if this is so, as will asking yourself questions such as:

- ○ Have you lost a few pounds?
- ○ Has your hair stopped falling out so much?
- ○ Are you on more even footing emotionally?
- ○ Do you wake up in the morning more refreshed and hopeful?

When you answer these questions, you will probably feel happier about your health than you have in a while. It's a wonderful thing to see yourself get better. But it can also be frustrating if all of your symptoms haven't completely gone away, or if you have developed other ones on top of the old. With this seemingly confusing pair of emotions, you will undoubtedly ask yourself what all this means.

What's going on?

Your body is going through a drastic adjustment. You have gone from inadequate thyroid hormone levels to supplementing what your thyroid makes with hormone that is supposed to put your metabolism back in balance, and all of your internal organs are getting used to the added boost they are getting from your new medication. You've felt some relief from this, but you're far from feeling 100 percent. This is because of altering your thyroid hormone levels and the impact that has on your body takes time.

Just how much depends on how severe your hypothyroidism was to begin with, what kind of medication you're on and how it reacts with your metabolism, and how careful you've been about sticking to your medication schedule and healthful regimen. Unfortunately, you can't speed up the effects of taking supplemental thyroid hormone, and you could do more harm than good by taking more supplement than you ultimately need. But you can make sure that you are doing everything possible to benefit from the dosage you are taking.

Taking stock of where you are

Sometimes, when I don't think a medication is working quickly enough, I get afraid that I'm wasting my time, money, and precious health. This fear works against my being at ease with my condition and weighs me down at a time when my emotions are already vulnerable.

Now that I keep a health journal and better monitor my progression through bouts with various symptoms, I can see that when I might think nothing is happening, something really is. My fear has subsided greatly, and I am more confident in my doctors and my ability to do the right thing for myself, even when thyroid fatigue wears me down. This helps me understand that I *am* doing something positive toward improving my condition, and it lessens my fear that I'll never feel better.

It also helps to remember that thyroid medication can bring a rush of energy and relief within weeks of when you begin taking it, but it can also work subtly. You might not notice that your metabolism is working better or that you are getting more restful sleep. Depression can still weigh you down, but it might not be as severe as it was a few weeks ago.

By looking over your health journal and reviewing where you were Day 1 and where you are now, you can better determine how well you are doing. You can also develop questions and comments for your doctor when you go back for your next examination and blood tests.

Another good thing to review right now is your "cycle history": the times when you have been caught up in good cycles, bad cycles, and what you've done about them. See if you can make any changes that might help you feel better, or that might alleviate more stress in your life. This applies especially to your relationships, which might have become strained when your condition was undiagnosed, or earlier in your treatment.

Friends in need, friends in deed

Sometimes, we don't know what affect our illness has on others until we begin to feel better. I think one of the main reasons for this is that when we are in pain, depressed, or otherwise feeling awful, we are, quite naturally, centered on ourselves. But as natural as this is, being self-centered can cause misunderstandings between loved ones, arguments, and sometimes complete rifts.

Now that you are feeling somewhat better, look at your relationships with your loved ones with new eyes. Have you unintentionally or on purpose caused pain? Are you needed by someone, but haven't stepped up to help? Do you wish you could be a better friend? Parent? Wife? Husband?

During these first months with hypothyroidism, you have acquired some amazing coping skills and are in the process of developing others. Use this knowledge to make your relationships what you want them to be. Look upon improving your future with your loved ones just as you do making yourself feel better. Having a strong support system, and being beloved as well as loved, is vital to your well-being, especially as you move forward with your life with hypothyroidism.

IN A SENTENCE:

> *Take stock of where you've been and where you are and develop a plan for improving areas of your life, especially relationships that might have suffered during your early days with hypothyroidism.*

learning

Frequently Asked Questions

SOMETIME AFTER the first two months of treatment, your doctor will ask you to come back for another examination and a series of blood tests. You will probably have a list of questions at this point. Here are some of the most frequently asked ones.

What should I expect at my follow-up examination?

Your follow-up examination will probably include the following:

- ○ A "weigh-in" (remember to take off your shoes!)
- ○ A blood pressure check and a check of your pulse, lungs, and heart.
- ○ A hand examination of the thyroid gland from the front and back.
- ○ A discussion of what medication you are on, the dosages and frequency, and how you feel, inside and out.

If you bring your list of medications and questions, you will be able to save time explaining everything and have more time to discuss what course of action should be taken. It helps if you *quantify* how you feel in relation to what you felt like on your first visit; even if you're not perfectly well, your doctor will want to know if you have sensed any improvement at all.

This second appointment is certainly the time to ask questions, too. Some of your most pressing questions might be:

○ Should I change my medication up or down in dosage?
○ Is there anything else I should be taking for my symptoms?
○ How do *you* [the doctor] think I'm doing?

Don't be surprised if your doctor doesn't give you definite answers right then. He or she will undoubtedly want to get the blood test results back before changing your medicine or dosage very much, if at all. Again, this is the time to be patient. Ask your doctor when he or she will call you with the test results (or when you can call your doctor's office for them). It is not unusual for doctors to make their calls after their last patient of the day, so try to be available in the evening, if that is when your doctor will call you.

After your doctor has reviewed your blood tests, ask your questions again. This time, you should have some answers and be able to enter the next phase of your treatment.

What is the prognosis for hypothyroidism?

If you are hypothyroid due to thyroid cancer and have had your thyroid gland removed, you should not experience much fluctuation in your thyroid hormone levels because you have to take supplemental thyroid hormone for all that you need. Your medication dosages and type could be stable for many years. If you are hypothyroid due to Hashimoto's thyroiditis, however, your thyroid levels might fluctuate as the autoimmune process flares and ebbs. Patients who have had Graves' disease might even experience times when they become hyperthyroid again, even if they have swung over to hypothyroidism. Once Hashimoto's thyroiditis is activated, however, eventually your thyroid gland will "burn itself out," and you will have to completely supplement the thyroid hormone your body needs.

Finding the right dosage and the right medication can take several months, if not years, as your gland's function ebbs and flows. Your doctor will gauge your medication needs by his or her examination, analysis of your lab results, and the information you provide about your symptoms and comfort level with your health. It is very important for you to be honest with your doctor throughout this process—and honest with yourself. Only through openness and trust can you work together toward a healthier you.

Should I take T_3?

This area of endocrinology is still very controversial. Some doctors feel that as long as your TSH is in the normal range, there is no need to look farther into your thyroid hormone balance, even if you are still symptomatic. Other physicians believe that there is benefit to examining whether raising T_3 levels even slightly will help the patient feel better and become more energetic and able to cope with life with hypothyroidism.

Patients who take T_3 often feel much better very quickly. But it is crucial that they really *need* the extra hormone, as opposed to wanting to have more energy. If someone gets too much T_3, he or she could develop serious heart problems, osteoporosis, or other complications, and/or become hyperthyroid. You should never self medicate, meaning you should never take more thyroid hormone, or a different combination of thyroid hormone, than what your doctor prescribes.

If your doctor does not want to explore the T_3 issue with you, it is perfectly all right to seek a second opinion from a reputable thyroid specialist. Also, make sure that you and your doctor have ruled out any autoimmune or other illnesses that might be combined with hypothyroidism and undermine your overall health.

Will I need to be hospitalized?

Hypothyroid patients rarely have to be hospitalized because of their thyroid disease. Thyroid cancer patients need hospitalization if they have their thyroid glands removed or undergo radiation therapy. Graves' disease patients and others who are hyperthyroid might also be hospitalized if their conditions get out of control, or if they have surgery to remove their thyroid glands. But hypothyroidism, although chronic and life-altering, does not usually lead to a hospital stay.

There are, of course, exceptions, especially if you have hypothyroidism and one or more other chronic illnesses. Here are some tips for surviving a hospital stay:

○ Know exactly why you are being hospitalized, how long you should be there, and if there are any complications that might arise to keep you there even longer. Also, find out the basic cost of your stay and figure this into your insurance and overall budget. Don't skimp on your healthcare, but do be prepared for whatever costs you might incur.

○ Prepare in advance by completing as much paperwork for the hospital as you can. Update your medical résumé and take several copies with you when you enter the hospital. Also, update your list of emergency contacts and make sure the hospital's records are up to date, too.

○ Notify your insurance company that you will be hospitalized and get preauthorization for the stay, procedures while you are there, and anything else that requires preauthorization.

○ Know who will be overseeing your care while you are in the hospital (sometimes there is a team of doctors and the line of communication and "command" might not be clear).

○ Appoint a family member or trusted friend as your "advocate" and make sure that person is familiar with the workings of the hospital. You want to make sure that, if you are unconscious or otherwise unable to advocate for yourself, you have someone you can trust who can "run interference" for you (or even do something as simple as get you a drink of water when you need it). If you don't have a loved one who can do this, think about hiring a nurse or other professional health advocate (ask your health insurance company or physician for referrals).

○ Ask to speak with the hospital chaplain or rabbi and benefit from his or her spiritual support in addition to the medical support you will get.

○ Try to keep track of all the medication, procedures, and other care that you receive and check your experience against the bills that you see after you are discharged. Watch out for charges for things that you never received and call your insurance company to clear up any errors.

○ When you leave the hospital, ask for a Release of Information form. About two weeks later, fax the completed form to the hospital and follow up with them to ensure that you get copies of all your records.

Above all, although this is difficult, try to maintain a positive attitude while you are in the hospital. Concentrate on getting better so you can get out—and do everything you can to make this happen.

If I already am hypothyroid, is there a possibility I might develop other illnesses?

Most people who are hypothyroid do not develop other autoimmune illnesses. However some seem to be "autoimmune disease magnets." I sometimes jokingly refer to myself as "the poster child for autoimmune illnesses" because I have so many different ones. (Have I mentioned yet that it's important to keep a sense of humor?)

Although autoimmune illness is not to be taken lightly, it doesn't help emotionally or physically to worry about coming down with something in addition to hypothyroidism. But it is important to know your body well enough to sense when something isn't right, and to tell your doctor if you think a symptom might be worse or if a new one appears. To do this, you need to rely on your own knowledge, a regular review of your symptoms at home and with your doctor, and, at times, assertiveness to get at the reason for something that doesn't seem right.

IN A SENTENCE:

> *Your follow-up examination is an important time for you to get answers to your questions, and familiarizing yourself with the ones that are most frequently asked can help you be better prepared to cope with your condition as well.*

MONTH **4**

living

Coping Strategies

FOR SOME people, supplemental thyroid medication *really* starts to work during this time. If this happens to you, this month could be terrific for you. There is nothing like experiencing the lifting of clouds caused by hypothyroidism—and seeing the brilliant sun shine through. All the things you hope to accomplish in your life beyond hypothyroidism could once again be within your reach.

But there are some things that might dim your happiness somewhat and cause you extreme frustration. For one thing, you are ever more aware that you will have to take medication daily—for the rest of your life—and be under regular, if not constant, medical care. You have a new identity: Besides being a mother, wife, husband, teacher, lawyer, or student, you are also a hypothyroid patient. Sometimes that sounds so depressing.

Also, you might be exploring the possibility of having other illnesses besides hypothyroidism. You might feel as though you've gone overboard into a sea of ill health and discomfort and not be able to find a way to get back onto the "life" boat.

A proactive attitude

By now, you know that the best reaction to your problems is to be proactive. You know that it's all right to be depressed, sad, or angry. But you also are aware that the best way to get to a better emotional and physical place is to take charge of your situation and work to make it better.

Some of the ways you can further help yourself now are:

○ Continue and grow in your meditation and/or prayer life so that you can better understand what's happening inside of you emotionally.
○ Look for ways to enhance your current healthcare by exploring some alternative therapies, with the guidance and support of your physician.
○ Spend more time in leisure activities and with loved ones to build even stronger relationships.
○ Attend a support group for hypothyroid patients and/or join a thyroid organization that has a strong education and patient support component.

"Diplomatic assertiveness"

Sometimes we can feel powerless in relation to our physician. After all, he or she has years of training and even more years of clinical experience. Our doctors have the power to prescribe medication, order tests, and diagnose illness. They sign our medical forms, approve our pursuit of disability status, and are the gatekeeper of one of the most important areas of our lives: our health.

But even with the difference in knowledge and expertise, there are times when we know better than anyone that something is wrong with our health. I experienced this first hand and have never forgotten.

In 1996, I began losing my hair. It pulled out of my head in fist-sized clumps and left smooth, round patches of scalp behind. The first time this happened, I was shocked and scared. I called my internist. He thought I was "stressed," and I did everything I could to feel less so. I took time off from work, pursued more leisure activities, practiced meditation and prayer even more than before. But my hair kept falling out. A few months later, my doctor asked me if, perhaps, I wasn't pulling my hair out myself (because of my stress).

Not a helpful question.

Something inside me clicked, and I knew I had to find out what was causing my hair loss and other puzzling symptoms.

It took me another several months to figure out just how to find answers. At the time, I had also been going to a dermatologist. During one of my many appointments, I asked her to run some blood work "because something else must be wrong." She didn't think I had anything to worry about, but agreed when I looked at her kindly, but firmly, and said, "Humor me."

Looking back, I think God must have been working overtime to get me to that point. I'd always trusted doctors to know better than I when something needed medical attention. But saying those two simple words enabled me to get blood tests that ultimately led to my being diagnosed with lupus and started on treatment.

The concept of "diplomatic assertiveness" was developed by Lisa Waldman, a clinical social worker and patient educator who often works with chronically ill patients. It enables a patient to use specific techniques to obtain appropriate and necessary medical care while preserving the doctor-patient relationship. In my case, being diplomatically assertive, as opposed to belligerent or defying, helped me continue to benefit from a doctor's ability to order tests and diagnose me. It also helped me learn how to speak up for myself when my inclination was to be intimidated by my doctors.

"You can use diplomatic assertiveness with your current doctor in order to enhance your rapport. For example, if you feel that your doctor isn't listening well or is rushing you through an appointment, you might say, 'Doctor, I know you must be very busy today, but I do have a few more concerns I would like to discuss with you before our meeting is over. I truly appreciate your patience.'

"You can also use diplomatic assertiveness if you feel you need to get a second opinion," says Waldman. "A lot of patients feel guilty about doing this, but when it comes to your health, you are the priority. You can maintain the integrity of your relationship with your current doctor by being honest and diplomatic. You might say, 'Because I'm dealing with a serious illness, I want as much information as I can get. I know you'll understand my seeking other opinions and I look forward to sharing what I've learned with you so we can move ahead.'"

"Diplomatic assertiveness can be applied to many different situations involving healthcare," says Waldman, "from hospital stays to lab visits. Decide what you need to know, or what you need to have done. Gently, but firmly, assert your need, always attempting to make the other person feel valued and helpful. Always give health professionals the benefit of the doubt by demonstrating to them that you understand their circumstances and limits. Make sure that you are polite, but if you don't get answers, keep asking and keep affirming your appreciation for the assistance, information, or service. And if someone dismisses your concerns, or is uncaring or rude, continue to be reasonable, but stand up for yourself. Remember, it is your body, your life. You deserve to get answers, and you deserve to be treated with respect and professional courtesy."

IN A SENTENCE:

> *Developing proactive coping strategies, including diplomatic assertiveness, will help you throughout your life and can also improve your sense of well-being.*

learning

Alternative Therapies and Practitioners

There is no herbal equivalent to supplemental thyroid hormone, so the hypothyroid patient must rely on his or her medical doctor for direct treatment for thyroid hormone imbalances. However there are some alternative therapies that have given hypothyroid sufferers relief from one or more of their symptoms. What you choose to do depends on:

○ Your level of comfort with certain therapies (some people don't like to be massaged, others are wary of taking herbs—and that's perfectly all right)
○ Your budget
○ The availability of products and practitioners in your area
○ Your doctor's recommendations and advice

Alternative therapies—an overview

In the U.S., the world of alternative therapies has expanded tremendously in recent years. To some people, the term "alternative" conjures up images of incense-burning gypsies and back-of-the-wagon elixir salesmen. However, today, the industry that encompasses herbal and dietary supplements, acupuncturists, chiropractors, hypnotherapists, and other practitioners has become sophisticated, organized, and more prevalent than ever before. Medical professionals are taking notice of the benefits of some therapies and are selectively including them in their patients' regimens. Medical schools are beginning to include some information about alternative treatments in their curriculum. And some insurance companies will consider coverage for some therapies.

Many of today's "alternative" treatments are based on folk or common traditions that predate modern, Western medicine. Others have been developed as adjuncts to treatments found in other cultures and medical traditions. Unfortunately, the modern scientific community has not produced a lot of hard data on many of the alternative products and services available today. This is partly due to lack of time and funds, and partly due to the still-present stigma against certain aspects of the alternative industry. For this reason, much of the "proof" of the efficacy of certain herbs and treatments remains anecdotal at best, and completely false at worst. The Food and Drug Administration does not regulate over-the-counter herbs and supplements, and as a result, potency and content often vary from batch to batch and from company to company. Regulation for alternative practitioners varies from state to state, with some states being more lenient than others. So it is difficult to compare "apples to apples" when you are looking for a reputable, competent practitioner, and sometimes it is hard to believe that a certain practitioner is interested in anything except making as much money as he or she can.

With all this in mind, many people do choose to take advantage of the alternatives available to them. Some suggestions for you to use when considering alternative therapies are:

○ Know what you need. Review your health journal, take stock of how you feel (and where you hurt), and talk with your doctor about exactly what symptom(s) you want to seek help for.

○ Know who you're looking for. Contact your state's health agency and find out what licensing requirements they insist upon for practitioners of the therapy you want. Contact the national accreditation agency for that discipline and get a list of referrals from them. Ask friends and other hypothyroid patients who they have gone to and who they like. Interview a few practitioners to see if you like their approaches.

○ Know what you're getting. If you are considering a dietary supplement or herbal preparation, find out exactly what is in it and how much is in it, and take all that information to your pharmacist and your physician for review. Do not trust products that list "secret" ingredients, or do not list all ingredients clearly on the package.

○ Know what you know. If you are confused by the advertising hype of a product, or if a practitioner refuses to explain exactly what he or she is doing and why, be cautious. In order to take full control of your health, you need to know exactly what treatment you are receiving, what it is supposed to do, and how long it will take to work.

○ Consider your budget. This is important because, although some insurance companies do cover certain treatments (acupuncture, for example), others do not. Alternative therapies can become very expensive, and you want to avoid financial stress.

○ Consider the source. Suggestions from your doctor are one thing, but sending away for a product advertised in a magazine is another. Be wary of "fads." Spend your money wisely.

Where to begin

One helpful source of basic information concerning alternative therapies is the Mayo Clinic's Web site (www.mayoclinic.com). Another is the National Center for Complementary and Alternative medicine. Both give patient-friendly definitions of the theories behind various practices, and, especially at the NCCA site, data from the latest scientific studies. In addition, your physician might be familiar with practitioners in your area, and other patients also might have contact information, as well as anecdotes about how particular treatments worked for them. Your state health and human services department, or medical services department, should be able to give you the licensing and/or certification requirements for specific practices. And if your insurance company covers alternative treatments, they might have referrals for you, too.

Some of the most common alternative and complementary practices include:

○ **Acupuncture.** The insertion of thin needles into your skin to facilitate the flow of energy (qi) necessary to treat pain and/or illness. Types of acupuncture include: Chinese (traditional), acupuncture where an electric current is used to heighten treatment, and a combination of Chinese and "electric." Several treatments might be needed before there is any relief from symptoms. If several weeks go by without relief, acupuncture is probably not going to help you. Some insurance companies cover acupuncture (check with your policy to see if this applies to you). Your doctor should be able to give you a referral to a reputable acupuncturist.

○ **Chiropractic care.** A chiropractor is trained to manipulate the spine in order to realign the body's skeletal structure and bring balance to a patient's health. Chiropractors are licensed by the states in which they practice and referrals can usually be obtained from your doctor or by contacting the American Chiropractic Association (www.amerchiro.org). You should make sure that you are not taking any medications that might cause adverse reactions to chiropractic care; prednisone, for example, can cause your bones to be more brittle and chiropractic manipulations can sometimes lead to bone breaks.

○ **Biofeedback.** This is a technology-based practice of attaching sensors to parts of your body that give you visual and audible feedback on how your body reacts to various stimuli. It promotes guided imagery, visualization, and body "retraining" to help patients better control their physical responses to stress. A trained physical therapist can sometimes conduct biofeedback sessions or recommend a competent practitioner.

○ **Hypnotherapy.** In many ways, hypnotherapy is similar to biofeedback in that it encourages retraining of habits, impulses, and some physical responses to tension and addictions, such as cigarette smoking and overeating. It can also be helpful in managing chronic pain. In hypnosis, you achieve a deep state of mental and physical relaxation. Some people do not want to do this, as it gives them a feeling of being out of control. As with any alternative therapy, you should be very careful about whom you select to conduct hypnosis sessions.

○ **Massage therapy.** This restful, relaxing therapy can be especially helpful if you react to tension and stress by tightening your muscles. As with any alternative practitioner, you have to feel comfortable with your massage therapist and trust his or her discretion and sensitivity to your needs. Licensed physical therapists sometimes also provide massage services, or they can recommend someone with whom they have worked.

○ **Herbs and vitamins.** It can be very confusing to know what to believe (and what to take) regarding the herbs, vitamins, and other supplements that are available on the market. Besides speaking with your doctor and a professional nutritionist, consulting certain publications and organizations for the latest information can be helpful. Each year in the autumn, for example, The Arthritis Foundation (www.arthritis.org) publishes a comprehensive list of popular herbs and also updates patients about what research has been done, what seems to be effective, and what doesn't. Also, before you supplement your diet with too many over-the-counter pills, be sure that you are getting as many nutrients as you can through the food that you eat.

○ **Yoga.** There are many kinds of yoga, ranging from physically challenging to a combination of meditation and more leisure stretches. Benefits from yoga include increasing your physical range of motion and mental and spiritual focus that can help you meditate and/or pray more effectively. Some video stores carry yoga tapes, which can be a good place to start, if you're completely unfamiliar with this discipline. Yoga schools are also helpful in matching you up with just the right style.

○ **Tai Chi.** This is another discipline, a form of martial arts, which combines physical and mental focus and movement. It is especially helpful to people who have trouble with their sense of balance (some of the movements and positions require you to stand on one foot or slowly move from position to position). There are Tai Chi schools and classes throughout the country, some connected with recreation centers.

IN A SENTENCE:

> *If you decide to pursue alternative therapies to help with one or more of your symptoms, it is a good idea to discuss what you want to do with your doctor, do in-depth research, and choose your options carefully.*

MONTH **5**

living

Hormones Wreaking Havoc

THERE'S A phrase that many women (and even some men) can relate to: "I'm so hormonal!"

There are times when there doesn't seem to be an explanation for the acute anxiety, anger, stress, or combination of cramps and malaise that assail us, especially at certain times of the month. "Hormonal" has become a code word for many women during the times that they feel their emotions and psyches are completely out of whack.

Is there, though, any truth behind this outburst of frustration and angst?

There could very well be.

During our child-bearing years, we women undergo hormonal surges and changes that accompany one of the most essential components of our sex: our ability to have children. First, we go through the "development" stage: puberty. Our bodies change seemingly before our eyes, while inside a process of hormone production occurs that triggers our first periods and every menstrual cycle thereafter. In adulthood, we undergo further change if we become pregnant. And as we mature past those child-bearing years, our hormonal balance changes once again as we travel through menopause.

Throughout all of these stages, our pituitary, hypothalamus, and thyroid glands are busy making the hormones that fuel each delicate event. When they are working properly, everything "hums." But when there is an imbalance, we can be affected greatly, sometimes severely.

"Feeling hormonal" can mean everything from being irritable in mid-menstrual cycle to developing a true, deep depression because of chemical imbalances within our bodies. Of course, these need to be weighed against our ability to cope with change, illness, and other challenges in life. But there could possibly be a component to your emotional state that is due to your thyroid's, or other glands' malfunction.

Investigating this possibility with your gynecologist and endocrinologist might yield some helpful information as to how you can adjust medication and/or lifestyle so that you are not so undermined by hormones gone out of control. There *are* things you can do to help yourself feel better, even in the most "hormonal" of times.

IN A SENTENCE:

> *The feeling of being "hormonal" might have some basis in truth, especially if your thyroid, pituitary, and/or hypothalamus is malfunctioning, and you should talk with your doctor about any symptoms you have to find out if something else is wrong.*

learning

What's Going on Inside Throughout the Month

THYROID HORMONES are one part of a complex system of hormones that circulate throughout the body and trigger a number of vital life processes. Hormones regulate follicle growth, reproduction, maturation, and gland function, among other activities. Whenever any hormone production is "off," that is, whenever there is too much or too little of any given hormone, glands and organs could malfunction, affecting your health and feeling of well-being. This is especially true for women during their menstrual cycle, which is regulated by a delicate balance of hormones.

The hypothalamus and the pituitary gland, which are so important to thyroid function, also play vital roles in a woman's monthly cycle and reproductive capability. The hypothalamus produces hormones that influence the pituitary gland to produce and release hormones, or not to release its hormones. The pituitary gland signals the reproductive organs to prepare for and carry out the ovulation cycle. If the thyroid gland is not producing enough hormone, or if the body is not converting enough T_4 into the active T_3, the hypothalamus and pituitary, which depend upon the active hormone to function properly, can be affected.

Some hypothyroid patients complain of excruciating PMS (premenstrual syndrome). Their symptoms might include severe cramping, emotional outbursts, depression, and extreme fatigue. Sometimes, too, periods disappear altogether, or become so sporadic that it is impossible to predict when they will occur. Usually, though, these symptoms improve when the supplemental thyroid hormone begins to work.

"Before I started my Synthroid, the PMS was so bad," says Pamela G., "that I couldn't leave the house. My periods were real bad, too. Now, everything's much better."

PMS or lack of periods can cause anxiety about what's happening inside your body. Also, if you want to get pregnant, having irregular periods or no periods can make that impossible and cause stress to your relationship with your partner, as well as to your self-image. (Infertility carries with it problems of its own, which is discussed in Month 7.)

It is very important that you discuss PMS symptoms and other menstrual problems with your doctor, perhaps with both your gynecologist and your endocrinologist. See if there might be an imbalance of estrogen that could contribute to your symptoms, and explore treatment possibilities with your physicians. Sometimes, birth control pills might help regulate your cycle and help you feel better. Or you might benefit from massage therapy, biofeedback, or another complementary treatment in conjunction with your thyroid hormone medication, at least until your thyroid hormone levels are more normal.

Relying on your stress management skills and practicing meditation and/or prayer can also help you lessen the tension of hormonal surges. So, too, can taking your concerns to your support group and discussing with others what they have done (you'd be surprised at how many hypothyroid patients have shared your problem).

Hormone replacement therapy (HRT), estrogen, and autoimmune disease

In recent months, there has been a lot of press about the dangers of hormone replacement therapy (HRT), particularly for women who have one or more autoimmune disease. This is due in part to a growing body of evidence that suggests that estrogen plays a significant role in the development of autoimmune disease. In numbers alone, this would seem to have a basis in fact; more than half of all people with autoimmune diseases are women. For example, more than 80 percent of the people who have systemic lupus erythematosus are women. There are similar statistics for other autoimmune illnesses, too, including Hashimoto's thyroiditis.

Many rheumatologists now recommend that lupus patients not take any HRT. Endocrinologists are not quite at that point with their Hashimoto's thyroiditis patients; however, it is a very good idea to discuss the pros and cons of HRT with your endocrinologist before proceeding with it. Take into account whether you have had Graves' disease and might be predisposed to developing osteoporosis. Consider that menopause is a natural part of aging and is finite in duration (hot flashes aren't forever). Also, understand that some research is ongoing, and answers might not be available just yet. Keep learning about the latest research in HRT and its effects on your body and spirit.

IN A SENTENCE:

> If you have significant PMS or other menstrual difficulties, discuss these with your doctor and see if there is an endocrine connection beyond thyroid hormone imbalance that might be affecting you.

Fear and Uncertainty in Intimacy

ONE OF the most sensitive topics for hypothyroid patients to cope with is intimacy. This is because of the psychological, emotional, and physical effects of hypothyroidism, and also because the patient has a huge "monster" to tend to apart from all other relationships. That monster, a chronic disease, never goes away and has to be constantly taken care of. It's no wonder, then, that in the first weeks and months following diagnosis, many hypothyroid patients find their intimate relationships strained.

If you have been experiencing a lack of libido, low self-esteem, and difficulty maintaining balance in your life, your relationships could be jeopardized. Some people coping with chronic illness even wonder if the man or woman they married, or if their partner, is really "the one" anymore. Sadly, the divorce rate among couples where one spouse has a chronic illness is above the national average.

Is it just your thyroid talking, or are you falling out of love?

There are many reasons why we fall in love. Common interests, "chemistry," shared values, like-minded goals—all of these figure into the romantic picture. But when a loved one becomes seemingly disinterested in intimacy and/or is moody and withdrawn, all of those wonderful reasons can suddenly be called into question.

Divorce is a drastic measure to dissolve a union between two people who once vowed to "love and cherish, in sickness and in health, 'til death . . ." So, too, is ending a long-term relationship or breaking up a shared household. Before taking a step of finality, it is helpful to review certain aspects of your life and the life you share with your loved one. Take into account:

○ Why you are together. What is your "basis for bonding"?

○ What specific problems need addressing between you?

○ How much of your problems are due to your worry over things you cannot control (such as the fact that you have a chronic illness) and how much is due to your health as a "work-in-progress"?

○ What life would be like without your loved one. Sometimes we don't fully appreciate someone until we imagine living without them.

○ How deep does your commitment go? Do you and your partner fully appreciate "in sickness and in health," or did you never take that seriously to begin with?

○ How much emphasis you put on intimacy and sex as the factor that keeps you together. A truly loving relationship is built on more than that, but it is also enhanced by it.

○ The course of your thyroid hormone treatment. Have you experienced an improvement in your libido since you started your medication?

Only you can decide when a relationship has fallen apart irreparably. But take time to determine if you need to divorce or break up. You might experience renewed interest in sex and intimacy as your medication begins to work more. Your moods might stabilize, too, so you can better relate to your loved one. And, if you are depressed, getting your thyroid hormones back into balance can make life much better—for you *and* the one you love.

Be careful

Sometimes, people react to their lack of libido by trying to force the issue. They become involved in sexual activities that they normally would not participate in simply because they want to see if they can push themselves to engage in sex. This kind of activity can lead to low self-esteem, embarrassment, and shame, and can expose you to sexually transmitted diseases and other harmful situations.

Talk with your doctor or counselor if you feel you are trying to engage in things that you really do not want to do. Be open and honest with yourself, and don't feel bad about saying no. It's your right, and if your partner cares about you, he or she will respect that.

IN A SENTENCE:

> Sometimes, it is easy to mistake a low libido for falling out of love; attention to intimacy in your relationship is important, but should be considered along with all other parts of a working, loving relationship.

learning

Help for Intimacy

WHEN YOU have a chronic illness, you need the full support of your family and friends in order to make it through the
rough first few months after diagnosis. Of course, you need
them going forward, too. But it is in the first six months that you
are trying to make sense of your life, your illness, and your
symptoms, and it is then, too, that you might experience your
greatest losses in activities and relationships.

Some hypothyroid patients lose interest in sex and intimate
activities with their partners, and this causes rifts and other
problems within their closest relationships. Those hypothyroid
patients who do not have a partner when they are diagnosed are
often hesitant to reach out and start relationships, because they
feel they are bringing an extra and unwanted burden with them:
a chronic illness.

But hypothyroidism does not preclude closeness between
husbands and wives, and it should not be the reason why people do not pursue long-lasting, loving relationships. In fact, having a chronic illness might enable two people to work harder at
finding more things in common than sex, and thus might
cement between them a greater, more resilient bond. Someone
who is hypothyroid might discover a true "gem" among potential partners, someone who accepts his or her illness and even

wants to help. Hypothyroidism causes physical symptoms that can be difficult to cope with, such as dry skin, vaginal dryness, and lost libido; and depression and fatigue are components of it, too. How do you promote intimacy and relationship-building when you don't feel like it, or when symptoms are so severe that you can't get out of bed?

Levels to love

There are many levels to loving someone. There is physical attraction, common goals, shared ideals and morals, spiritual bonding, geographic proximity, and willingness to compromise and accommodate the other person in times of need. Each of these levels has, within it, different sublevels, or areas that make up the whole. And at any given time, one of these levels might be more predominant in the relationship than another. This includes the intimacy involved in relating to one another physically, as well as to the other levels.

In a relationship, especially one that is long-lived, physical attraction can increase and decrease. Life, aging, stress, and illness play a part in this. How you and your partner approach your physical relationship is important, and the earlier you work out a game plan for times when one or the other of you is less interested, the better.

"Sex is great and fine, but I don't always want it because I'm tired," says Pamela G. "Your spouse needs to understand that it's not him, but you're just tired. You have to have good communication with your spouse."

Other helpful ways to work together are:

○ Explore ways that you can enjoy physical closeness without engaging in fully consummated sex.
○ Learn to love the changes that have taken place with your loved one's appearance or focus on an aspect, such as eye color or smile, that is less changeable.
○ Go back to "dating" to rekindle the original attraction and excitement that was there earlier in your relationship.
○ Laugh together.
○ Recognize that hypothyroidism can be treated with medication and problems with intimacy can be alleviated as thyroid hormone levels increase. Be patient, be hopeful.

○ Try not to be obsessive about the changes in your or your partner's libido and/or interest. The more you push it, the more it will cause pain and anxiety between you.

Physical symptoms

A good dermatologist can help you find a skin lotion or ointment that can take the itch out of your dry skin, as well as restore some moisture to it. K-Y Jelly or another vaginal lubricant can help with dryness (your gynecologist can suggest something). Muscle and joint pain can be eased a bit if you take a warm bath and do stretches before you approach your husband or wife intimately. Learning massage techniques can be a good way to bring a healing touch to your relationship. And working together to find a physical routine that satisfies both of you is important, too.

Lidia Q. says, "My husband is a hottie, but it doesn't always register below. We've found a pattern, a compromise. Most married couples have to do that."

And if your husband wants to have sex, but your hypothyroidism is preventing you from looking forward to it as much as he is?

"It's not horrible," says Lidia Q. "It's not like root canal. You like the fact that they're happy. Whatever your problem is, you have to work around it."

Dating and hypothyroidism

In the first few months after diagnosis, if you aren't dating someone or you aren't married, you might not feel like being very sociable. That's all right. There will be time for getting back into the dating scene when you start to feel better. When you do decide to jump into the "pool," here are some excellent traits to look for in someone to date:

○ Compassion and understanding
○ Willingness to learn about your condition
○ A helpful nature, but not smothering
○ Ability to express interest in other parts of your life besides your illness
○ Follow-through on encouraging you to do things that are healthful
○ A good, healthy attitude toward life
○ Ability to care for him- or herself

Don't feel as though you have to tell the person you date about your illness the first time you meet. There will be time enough to tell the man or woman you're seeing about your chronic illness. On the first few meetings, observe his or her response to life, your conversations, and learn as much about him or her as you can. You want to be sure that whomever you date will be understanding of your illness, but you should wait until a time in your relationship when you feel comfortable telling him or her about it. Hypothyroidism is a big part of your life, but it's not the only thing. You want to find overall compatibility in order to forge a relationship that will last.

Toxic relationships

In each of our lives, there have been or are people who do not uplift us, but rather weigh us down. These might be spouses, significant others, family members, friends, or acquaintances. Treating your personal life as you would your physical health, it is important to look upon relationships as things that should be healthful and rejuvenating, as well as mutually important and supportive.

Toxic relationships are those that overall do not help us but rather hinder us from realizing the full potential of our personal selves. They might be:

- ○ Argumentative
- ○ One-sided
- ○ Cloying
- ○ Jealous
- ○ Petty
- ○ Physically unhealthful
- ○ Dangerous
- ○ Selfish
- ○ Built on only superficial needs and desires

Having a chronic illness gives us the opportunity to examine the relationships in our lives and weed out those that are not healthful for ourselves or, perhaps, for the other person involved. There are times when we cannot completely separate ourselves from toxic individuals; family members are sometimes there to stay. But we can work out ways to distance ourselves enough from them so that their toxicity does not pollute our lives, hearts, spirits, and souls. It can be difficult to say good-bye. But realistically, sometimes we can only move along our healing path when we do.

IN A SENTENCE:

> *There are remedies for some of the physical symptoms of hypothyroidism that prevent you from desiring intimacy with your partner, and there are certain characteristics you can look for in another person that will help you find a nurturing, healthful relationship.*

HALF-YEAR MILESTONE

It's been six months, and, although sometimes it seems as if it's been six years, you are making great progress. During these few short months you've:

○ DEVELOPED A FRAME OF REFERENCE FOR QUESTIONS YOU NEED TO ASK AND ANSWERS YOU RECEIVE, AS WELL AS INFORMATION THAT YOU FIND REGARDING YOUR HEALTH AND WELL-BEING.

○ GAINED TREMENDOUS INSIGHT INTO YOUR ABILITY TO HANDLE STRESS ON THE JOB AND AT HOME, AND YOU'VE TAKEN STEPS TO BE EVEN BETTER AT IT.

○ ORGANIZED YOUR LIFE TO ACCOMMODATE YOUR ILLNESS WHILE STILL KEEPING THE QUALITY OF YOUR PURSUITS AND INTEGRITY OF YOUR RELATIONSHIPS.

○ SET OUT A FINANCIAL GAME PLAN FOR TAKING CARE OF YOUR HEALTH AND YOUR OTHER RESPONSIBILITIES—AND PROVIDED FOR LEISURE ACTIVITIES, TOO.

○ WORKED WITH YOUR DOCTOR TO DETER-MINE IF THERE IS ANY OTHER HEALTH issue besides hypothyroidism that you need to address.

- Reached out to loved ones, firmly cemented those relationships that are truly important, and reviewed those that are troubled or "toxic."

- Begun to work with your husband, wife, or partner to find ways to promote your relationship even when you do not feel like being intimate.

Family Life

HAVING A family is one of the most marvelous parts of being human. Having a family *and* having a chronic illness is a challenge, but certainly one worth facing. Loved ones can bring so much support and comfort to you in your suffering (and joy and love) that you benefit more from maintaining your nurturing relationships than severing them.

Still, it is difficult to be a 100 percent parent when you are fatigued, an attentive spouse when your brain is foggy, or a cheerleader for the whole family when you suffer from depression. The demands of being a mom or dad, husband or wife can be overwhelming when you don't feel well.

How can you continue to be a good, loving family member when you are barely able to move through each day with hypothyroidism?

○ *Recognize your limits.* Everyone has them, but sometimes, if we have to take care of small children or be active with our spouse, we push our own needs into the background. This is the sign of being a loving person, but it can also damage the progress you're trying to make to help yourself feel better. Take stock of what you can and can't do. Acknowledge where your boundaries are. Communicate them in love and care, explaining that you want to feel better so that you can truly participate in your loved ones' lives.

○ *Be honest with yourself and your loved ones.* Don't hide behind your illness, but rather discern whether you don't feel like being an active part of the family for reasons other than hypothyroidism. Seek counseling or medical attention to get at the root of what your other issues might be, and follow through with the treatment or therapy that you and your doctor decide upon.

○ *Teach your children.* Use your illness as a valuable lesson in life for your children. Even the youngest child can probably understand that their mommy or daddy doesn't feel well. Assure your children that you will feel better soon, and, whenever appropriate, ask him or her for assistance in even the smallest of chores so that they can become used to helping instead of fearing illness.

○ *Laugh together.* Children and spouses pick up the subtlest of cues from one another. Often, the habits developed at an early age become lifelong traits. Learning how to have an appropriate sense of humor is an important lesson and coping technique with any chronic illness. Not that hypothyroidism is funny, but some of the things that come from it can be. For example, instead of being hard on yourself for forgetting to do something, laugh about it being "that brain fog again."

○ *Have a support system.* The strongest of families will be even stronger if its members have support from extended family members, friends, a faith community and/or medical professionals. Sometimes, counseling can help resolve problems that arise due to one family member's chronic illness.

IN A SENTENCE:

A family is a wonderful gift to all involved, and the more you nurture your own health and the well-being of your family, the more you will benefit from its love, nurturing, and strength.

learning

Pregnancy and Parenthood

ADEQUATE THYROID hormone is vital to conceiving children and carrying them to term. It is also supremely important to the proper development of the unborn child and the newborn. Because of this, monitoring thyroid function should be part of a woman's preparation if she wants to become pregnant, and part of her healthcare from then onward. Also, in the U.S., all newborns are tested for their thyroid function and hormone levels; this practice is becoming common in other parts of the world, too.

Thyroid hormone and fertility

For the purposes of this discussion, I'm going to use the definition of infertility presented by Daniel Glinoer, M.D., Ph.D., in his keynote clinical address at the seventy-fourth annual meeting of the American Thyroid Association. According to Dr. Glinoer, "Infertility is defined as the absence of pregnancy after one year of unprotected sex."[1] The statistics presented by Dr. Glinoer are as follows:

○ Infertility affects 10 to 15 percent of couples
○ Thirty-five percent of cases of infertility are due to the female
○ Thirty percent of cases of infertility are due to the male
○ Fifteen percent of cases of infertility are due to both the female and male
○ Twenty percent of cases of infertility are due to ideopathic causes (that is, its causes are unknown)[2]

There seems to be a correlation between women who miscarry and women who carry the thyroid antibodies and who are **euthyroid** (that is, they have a normal TSH and a normal free T_4). The reason for this association cannot be fully explained, however there are some hunches. Perhaps, according to Dr. Glinoer, there is a generalized immune disregulation that causes the miscarriages. Or there could be "local," subclinical hypothyroidism that is not easily detected by the usual tests and examinations. The third hypothesis is that there is an indirect effect of older age; many of the women who experience miscarriage and who have thyroid antibodies are in their late thirties and forties.

Although it might seem a simple thing to do, sometimes fertility specialists overlook the thyroid, a fundamental aspect of a woman's health, and, instead, focus on more elaborate reasons for infertility. Before spending thousands of dollars on costly and imperfect fertility studies and treatments, the first thing a woman who has trouble conceiving should do is have her thyroid levels (hormones and antibodies) checked. Besides the supposed effect of the thyroid antibodies on fertility, having low thyroid hormone levels can prevent pregnancy because it can disrupt the menstrual cycle, as well as interfere with the adhesion of the fertilized egg and sperm to the uterine wall.

Thyroid and pregnancy

If a woman is hypothyroid, there is potential risk to both her and her unborn child. Being hypothyroid can increase the rate of obstetrical complications, such as premature birth, and postpartum hypothyroidism and postpartum depression. Hypothyroidism in the mother can also have a direct and negative impact on the unborn child because it can reduce the transfer of adequate thyroid hormone from the mother through the placenta to the fetus. Treating hypothyroidism before pregnancy can improve the chances of a woman becoming pregnant (if hypothyroidism has been causing infertility) and also improve her ability to carry her pregnancy to term. A good endocrinologist will work with the rest of the medical team to ensure that all thyroid hormone levels are kept in the appropriate ranges.

It is usually all right to continue taking your supplemental thyroid hormone throughout pregnancy, although the dosages might need to be adjusted up or down. Again, work with your endocrinologist and gynecologist to do what is right for you and your child.

Thyroid hormone and baby development

In the first trimester, the fetus is completely dependent upon the mother for all thyroid hormone. In the second trimester, the fetus's thyroid begins to function and, later, to produce thyroid hormone. But throughout the rest of gestation, thyroid hormone levels produced by the fetus do not exceed 50 percent of what the unborn child needs to develop normally. A lack of adequate thyroid hormone can lead to developmental problems, including lower IQ (which can translate into behavioral problems and difficulty learning) and, in the most extreme cases, produce cretenism.

Proper monitoring of the mother's thyroid hormone throughout her pregnancy can provide vital information to her and her physician about what, if any, measures need to be taken to increase the amount of thyroid hormone available to her and to her unborn child. In the U.S., newborn babies' thyroid function is checked as a matter of course immediately following birth to make sure that there are no problems. They should also be checked if a child's development seems slow or stunted in any way, as thyroid problems can occur in the days, weeks, and years afterward, too.

Thyroid hormone and postpartum depression

According to the Thyroid Foundation of America, thyroid problems tend to develop in the mother two to three months after delivery. Also, if you have had thyroid changes related to one pregnancy, you'll probably have them in subsequent ones, too.[3]

Is there any way to tell what will happen after pregnancy? One test might be a good indicator. Basil Rapoport, M.B., a research thyroidologist, says,

"Women who have the TPO antibodies (TPO-Ab) might be at a 30 percent higher risk for developing hypothyroidism and postpartum depression."

The American Association of Clinical Endocrinologists (AACE) also accepts the importance of the TPO-Ab test. In their recommended guidelines for monitoring thyroid levels during pregnancy, they say, "Pregnant women who have high TPO-Ab titers but normal serum thyrotropin levels should undergo careful postpartum and long-term follow-up because of the high probability of subsequent clinical hypothyroidism."[4]

It is important to remember that help *is* available to you if you are hypothyroid *and* suffer from postpartum depression. By working closely with your entire medical team you will be able to successfully get through it.

The fear of passing it along

Although there seems to be a genetic component to developing autoimmune illness and thyroid disease specifically, the connection is still unclear. Of the studies that have been done thus far, there doesn't seem to be any *assurance* that a mother who has thyroid antibodies will pass them along to her child, nor is there any proof that if you have thyroid disease, your children will have it, too.

It is natural to want the best for your children, and it is also natural to be afraid that you might give them the chronic illness that has gripped you. But because there is no definitive way to tell whether you *will* pass it along, fearing that you will might cause you to make a decision not to have children, which can, in turn, lead to a less joyful, wonderful family life.

As you well know, there are remedies for many of the symptoms that you suffer from, and there is medication to replace the thyroid hormone your gland isn't able to make. The same remedies, and probably many more, will be available to your children should they need them. Your awareness of thyroid disease and your "patient sophistication" will be an asset to them, even if they don't develop a thyroid problem. You will be able to teach them about a very important part of life—having empathy for someone who is ill—and inspire them through your example.

Before you decide not to have children, weigh the consequences very carefully and with hope and openness to the positives, as well as the potential negatives.

Birth control

There is really no contraindication between hypothyroidism and birth control pills (oral contraception). However, you should make sure that you are receiving your medication through a competent physician who understands your personal health picture and all the medication you are taking. If you want to practice "natural" birth control (the rhythm method, for example), you might have to rethink it if your hypothyroidism is still very symptomatic; low thyroid hormone levels can interfere with the menstrual cycle and make it difficult to tell when you are or are not fertile.

Options to pregnancy

Today, more than ever, there are many options open to couples (or single people) who want to have children but cannot conceive or carry pregnancy to term. These options include adoption, foster parenting, and surrogate parenting.

Also, there are many children in our communities and in the world at large who crave a family or the influence and care of concerned, responsible adults. If direct parenting is not possible for you, consider working closely with children's organizations or being a big brother or big sister. You can still make a significant difference in a child or children's lives, and bring fulfillment to your own, too.

IN A SENTENCE:

> *Hypothyroidism can have an effect on the mother and child, so it is very important that you seek competent medical monitoring before, during, and after pregnancy for both yourself and your baby.*

MONTH 8

living

Relationships: What Others Can Do

DURING THESE past few months, you've undoubtedly heard more than one loved one ask, "What can I do for you?" Perhaps you've had answers for them. But perhaps you've been at a loss as to what they can actually do.

This is quite natural. Coping with a chronic illness is a very lonely pursuit. It is up to you to identify and cope with your symptoms, to take your medication, and make and keep your doctor's and lab appointments. You need to understand your body and your condition, and you need to control what you eat, how much exercise you get, and other important health-related things in your life.

Beyond what you have to do for yourself, you know that there are things over which you, your doctors, and your loved ones have no control. You can't control that you became hypothyroid. You can't control the course that the disease will take, or whether you will develop other autoimmune illnesses on top of the one you have. You can't control the cost of medication, the price of lab tests and doctor's visits, nor can you really control the cost that the disease brings into your life and that of your loved ones.

But as you realize this, know, too, that part of being an *excellent* patient is being a *proactive* patient. For you to feel better, you need to support your health—and let others help you as you do so. And of course, because loving and being loved is a two-way street, you need to find ways to be a friend or a loved one, in return.

Much of this Living section is actually aimed at the people who care for and about you. You might like to read through this section together, and talk about what might apply (or what might not) to your particular situation. The ideas and tips are meant to spark thought and discussion between you and your loved ones, to help you all understand that fostering healthy relationships is vital to living a healthy life.

The tangible things

When someone asks you, the patient, how they can help, you might immediately think of tangible, concrete things that could be done. Helping with chores, driving the car pool, picking up groceries, taking on a pending project at work—all are practical things that someone might step in and do if you are too tired or otherwise too symptomatic to do them successfully yourself. It is helpful if you write a list of things that someone else could do and keep it handy for the times when you are in need of assistance. That way, you won't put yourself under undo stress to think of something.

Other concrete things that one might do don't necessarily relate to accomplishing a task or chore, but they do provide support. These include:

- ○ Taking a walk or running together
- ○ Meditating or praying together
- ○ Going out to a movie or museum and "just being" together
- ○ Reading the same book and then talking about what you've read
- ○ Engaging in active communication.

Active communication for the patient and loved one

I've heard many married couples say that they know just what the other person is thinking before they even speak. This is remarkable, and often happens. However, there are times when our loved ones have no clue what we need unless we speak up. We shouldn't fault them for not having a "second sight" or intuition regarding our needs or how we feel; no one is that all-knowing. We need to engage in active communication so that we are clear about our perspective and understand our loved one's, too.

Active communication is based upon a simple premise: *Two-way talking, two-way listening*. It is most effective when both people engaged in the communication are calm, focused, and desirous of achieving a new level of understanding between them. It is based upon mutual respect, affection, and trust.

Two-way talking occurs when two people involved in a discussion express simply and fully what is in their hearts and minds. They do not seek to persuade each other to change their opinions, biases, or fears. Rather, each states his or her "case" and allows the other person to formulate opinions and feelings about what is said. For example, if your husband wants you to stop volunteering at school because he thinks you're too frazzled, he might say, "I feel bad for you, honey. I feel like you're going to hurt yourself and your health by keeping so busy." Or, if you are particularly irritable because pain is overwhelming you, you might tell your parent, "I'm in such pain that I can't think straight, and I'm probably saying things that are hurtful to you."

Once someone has spoken, in active communication, the listener takes time to hear the words and feel the emotion behind them. In this way, your response to your husband might not be defensive, so much as compassionate, and your spouse might develop insight into what you're going through that he or she normally would not achieve.

Active communication takes time to develop. It is so easy to be *reactive* to the things that people say, especially when spoken in the heat of the emotional moment. But if put into practice, active communication can foster more empathy, understanding, and cooperation between loved ones and take some of the edge off of not knowing what to do for the people or person in their lives that is in pain.

Disappointments

Often, as we continue living with a chronic illness, there will be a person or persons who won't understand the ongoing nature of our condition. They'll expect us to be well after a week, a month, or two months. "Aren't you in remission yet?" they'll ask. Or, worse, "But you *look* great. I don't think your doctor knows what she's talking about, telling you you still have to take medication."

Part of how these people react to us is due to ignorance, but part of it can also be due to a disappointment in the realization that we are human and sometimes we get sick—very sick. People might be disappointed in us (hey, aren't we disappointed in ourselves, sometimes, too?).

Tips from One Who Knows
to Other Caregivers

MY mother has been beside me each time I've received a diagnosis of another disease. Here are her suggestions about how a loved one might view the patient's illness, as well as some suggestions for coping:

"You have to be very sensitive to the person when he or she receives a diagnosis of a chronic, serious illness. The least helpful reactions are those that drive the person away from you. These include:

○ Being in denial ('Are you sure?')

○ Offering no support ('Many people have the same trouble.')

○ Being a pseudo-doctor ('Oh, I know all about that. Let *me* tell you . . .')

○ Exhibiting anger

More helpful responses include:

○ Offering sympathy ('I'm sorry. Is there anything I can do?')

○ Relaying family history to validate the patient ('You know, your grandmother had the same thing.')

○ Showing concern ('How do you feel?')

○ Making simple inquiries ('How serious is your condition? What do you need to do to treat it?')

She adds, "Be there for the person. It's as simple as that."

When a loved one falls from a pedestal, so to speak, relationships that weren't that strong to begin with can fall apart. If you used to have enough energy for three people, your friends (or friend) might not be able to take your sudden "plunge to earth." Sometimes, all it takes is a diagnosis of a chronic illness to make people turn away, no longer call, or sever the relationship.

If someone you love starts to pull away, try to talk with him or her about what is making them do that. See if there is some level of understanding or knowledge that they need to be able to overcome their misgivings. Engage in active communication, where you truly listen to one another and try to meet halfway. But also accept that there will be some people who don't have the depth of spirit or character to maintain a friendship or relationship when

Coping Skills for Loved Ones

IF someone you love is ill, you might want to do everything for that person to the detriment of your own health and well-being. In love and understanding, strive to keep your own life in balance and operating smoothly:

○ Maintain your own health, taking care that you get enough sleep, rest, and exercise, and that you eat properly.

○ Get regular health check-ups, apart from the doctor's visits you go to with your loved one.

○ Cultivate outside friends and interests to keep your mind and enthusiasm fresh.

○ Join a support group for "caring others," people who care for and about loved ones who are chronically ill (contact the Thyroid Foundation of America or other patient organization for further information).

○ Nurture your spiritual life, enhance your quiet time with plenty of prayer, meditation, or introspection to find a deep, abiding peace.

○ Find a way to communicate with your loved one even when he or she is extremely fatigued or in pain; benefit from just *being* together and take comfort in the presence of your relationship.

it hits difficult waters. Find the strength within you to let go, and focus on relationships that are joyous, nurturing, and deep enough to bring you happiness and fulfillment throughout the rest of your life.

IN A SENTENCE:

Loved ones usually want to help, and giving them tangible ways to do so can foster greater understanding and a stronger bond among everyone involved.

learning

Relationships:
What You Can Do

THE IMPORTANT role of loved ones in our lives cannot be overstated. They are the glue that keeps us together, engaged in the world and able to battle our disease in all of its many facets. We often marvel at what it is that gives them the ability to give us such support, or what it is that makes them stick with us when others turn away.

And perhaps most important, we reflect upon what we can do to help them achieve their dreams, be a part of their lives, and give back to them what they give to us.

Our personal heroes

True heroes don't often think of themselves as heroic. Firemen who rush into burning buildings, mothers who shield their children from harm, ordinary people who do extraordinary things—most would probably say that they were just doing "what was right," "what was instinctive." But that doesn't take away from their accomplishments, nor does it diminish the value that they bring to our lives and everyone they come in contact with.

The heroes in our lives are those who take extra time and effort to talk with us, support us, and do the things that we're too weak or sick to do ourselves. They are also our cheerleaders and "coaches," encouraging us to stretch our boundaries when we are on the verge of giving up. They do things out of love, out of the honor of a commitment they have made, and the joy that comes from being linked with us—what a marvelous, wondrous gift it is to have people like this in our lives!

It helps to remember that our heroes need help and support, too. Here are a few things to keep in mind:

- ○ Encourage your loved ones to get proper healthcare and take care of themselves.
- ○ Respect your loved ones' need for activities, friends, and quiet time apart from you.
- ○ Express your thanks for the things that your loved ones do for you—don't take their actions or affection for granted.
- ○ Assist your loved ones to achieve their full potential; learn about what's important to them and try to be supportive along the way.
- ○ Know when to stay close and when to stand back, nurturing a fluid, restful relationship among you.
- ○ Pray for your heroic loved ones or meditate on their success, health, and happiness.
- ○ Appreciate the small things, as well as the large things, about your relationships, and treasure them in your "memory album."

IN A SENTENCE:

Identify the heroes in your life and take extra effort to nurture them and love them just as they love and nurture you.

Leisure Time

ALTHOUGH YOU have a chronic illness, there should be no reason why you have to put aside activities that you enjoy because of it. To be sure, fatigue can interfere with your ability to do many things in one day, so you might find that during the work week you won't have time for hobbies. And physical pain or other symptoms might mean that you will have to plan vacations and travel more prudently. But you don't have to give up these things altogether.

Depression

If you are depressed, your desire to engage in outside activities might be diminished considerably. If you aren't very active, or don't have much contact with a supportive group of friends and loved ones, you could become even more despondent. Be candid with your doctor and yourself about how you feel and try to work out a plan so that you can tackle your depression and become more interested in your life and activities. Start by taking small steps toward goals you want to achieve, and keep track of your progress in your health journal, reviewing your success and building upon it as you proceed.

Fear

Perhaps you hesitate to become involved in leisure activities because you are afraid of the impact they will have on your fragile health. This is very common, especially during the first year of coping with a new and sometimes confounding illness. Accept your fear, but also explore ways that you can respond to your trepidation with concrete and comforting solutions.

For example:

○ Know your boundaries (what you can and can't do physically). Accept them and choose activities that are within your current capabilities and desires.

○ Talk to other people who have chronic illness and who have done what you want to do. Ask them what they did to overcome their fear and make the activity healthful for them.

○ Familiarize yourself with the place where the activity is to occur (arena, classroom, art center, or athletic venue). Explore the environs so you are relaxed about being there and know what to expect.

○ Engage in the activity with a trusted friend or family member.

○ Discuss what you want to do with your doctor and ask him or her for pointers about how to approach it.

IN A SENTENCE:

Fear and depression can cause us to pull back from activities we ordinarily would find pleasure in, but it is possible to overcome them by working honestly with ourselves, our medical team, and our loved ones.

learning

Making Your Dreams Come True

WITH CAREFUL planning and recognition of the special needs you have because you have a chronic illness, you should be able to participate in the leisure activities you've always dreamed about (or have already enjoyed). Here are some tips on some of the most popular areas of enjoyment to give you an idea of how to approach them.

Travel

Traveling with a chronic illness is sometimes like moving along with an unseen, very unwelcome partner. You have to pack extra things (medications, list of emergency contacts, prescriptions), plan your schedule more carefully (maybe sightseeing isn't a good idea on the first day of your arrival in London), and overcome the fear and uncertainty of leaving your support system, doctors, and comfortable home behind.

In today's world, traveling is an uncomfortable business even for the healthiest person. Delays at the airport, extra security screening, and other complications make it a test for patience, endurance, and common sense. When you add your "invisible companion," your hypothyroidism, to the mix, you can immediately see that traveling can be troublesome. So, you have to plan accordingly, eliminating as much anticipated stress as possible and developing a good attitude toward the unexpected stresses that might occur.

○ **Carry extra insurance.** Whether you are traveling outside or within the U.S., you should invest in two kinds of travel insurance: trip cancelation insurance, and medical evacuation and repatriation insurance. The first kind will cover you if you have to cancel the trip because of illness, or if the trip is canceled in part or in whole because of the bankruptcy of the travel company or other problem. You can purchase this insurance from your travel agent, and it is usually very reasonably priced. Medical evacuation and repatriation insurance covers you if you fall ill while traveling and need to go back home for medical treatment. One company, MedJet (www. medjetassistance.com), employs a fleet of medically equipped and staffed airplanes and will pick you up wherever you are and fly you back to your home hospital and medical team. Their fee covers you for a full year, and will provide you with their services in the U.S. or abroad. This is an excellent option and can give you tremendous peace of mind, especially if you are traveling a long distance to a place where healthcare might be "iffy" at best.

○ **Know before you go.** Do as much research as you can on where you are going and how you will get there. Find prudent shortcuts and tips in books such as Peter Greenberg's (*The Travel Detective* and *Flight Crew Confidential*). Contact the local visitor's bureau where you are going and ask for their guidance in planning a stress-free visit.

○ **Packing.** Today, airlines allow each passenger one carry-on, and all other luggage must be checked in. You should *never* put your medication or other health-related necessity in your check-in baggage, but rather should carry it onto the plane with you. Leave your meds in their pharmacy-provided vials so that you can show the security guards that the prescriptions are yours. Also carry an extra copy of your prescriptions and a note from your doctor explaining your condition for extra protection.

○ **Medical Identification Tag.** Anyone who is taking medication should have a bracelet, necklace, or other means of identification that paramedics would find immediately if they are injured and/or unconscious. MedicAlert (www.medicalert.com) is one company that you may subscribe to. For an annual fee, you receive a bracelet or necklace that has your name, pertinent health conditions or medication allergies, your identification number, and a toll-free telephone number. Paramedics or other emergency personnel can call the telephone number, which is available twenty-four hours a day, seven days a week, and be advised of your primary care physician, emergency contact, and other health information that can have an impact on the type or degree of treatment you should receive.

○ **Physician referrals.** Contact the thyroid organization where you will be and/or ask your doctor for a referral to a physician there, in case you need medical attention.

○ **Ask for help.** You might hesitate to take advantage of the help available at airports, train stations, and other travel venues, but it is there for you. Skycaps can provide you with baggage assistance, and airport personnel can obtain a wheelchair for you if you're too fatigued to navigate the long and crowded airport terminals. Some airports have handicapped lounges, where you can receive special assistance with your flight arrangements (very handy, especially at holiday time). And hotels usually have accommodations for people with a myriad of physical requirements. To find out what's available for you when you decide to travel, all you have to do is ask!

Sports and other physical activities

Unless you are severely hypothyroid and have developed heart complications, there should be no restrictions on your ability to participate in sports, hiking, sailing, or any other physical activity. To be on the safe side, you might want to discuss with your doctor what you'd like to do and see if you need to do any pre-training to minimize the risk of overextending or injuring yourself. But beyond prudent precautions, recreational exercise is an excellent way to become and stay fit.

Hobbies and pastimes

When you have a chronic illness and it affects your ability to be productive, you can start to feel "useless." Having a hobby or other leisure activity can help you overcome your frustration at not being able to keep yourself as active as you once were. It can also be a good way to meet others with like-minded interests, and can enable you to focus on something other than your illness (sometimes, we become too self-centered, and this can create more problems than relief).

If you are especially fatigued, or your symptoms and possibly other illnesses prevent you from doing anything too strenuous, consider more sedentary activities that can challenge your mind and emotions. Some of these might be:

- Drawing, painting, writing, or pottery
- Stamp, coin, or watch collecting
- Doll and teddy bear making
- Jewelry, gems, and gemology
- Knitting, crocheting, sewing, embroidery, or needlepoint
- Model-building and woodworking
- Armchair traveling
- Calligraphy or origami
- Ham radio operating

Making it happen

Whenever I try to achieve something and am not feeling well, I use the following formula to give myself a framework to succeed:

Prioritize. I decide what is essential, important, and not-so-important about the things that I want to do and the things that I have to do.

Plan. Using a timeline and a good sense of what I'm physically capable of doing, I draw up a schedule for how I'd like my activities to proceed. I keep in mind that my health might delay things at any moment, but I can forge ahead whenever I can.

Practice. Achieving anything worthwhile doesn't happen overnight. It takes practice and, especially with a chronic illness, stopping and starting. Rather than thinking about not being able to finish something as a *failure*, I think about it as *a practice attempt* and, if it's something I really want to do, I keep at it until I can see it through to the end.

Patience. There will be times when health will intervene, when I won't be able to accomplish my goals and dreams. But I know that these setbacks are only temporary; just as there are downtimes, there are upswings. Realizing this, and riding out the tough times with patience, is vital to being ready to *enjoy life* when I'm feeling better.

IN A SENTENCE:

> *Engaging in leisure activities is important to overall well-being, and though there may be times when your health won't allow you to do them, with careful planning and patience, you should be able to do things you truly enjoy.*

living

Looking Ahead in Health

MANY PEOPLE are diagnosed with hypothyroidism when they are young—in their thirties and forties. As they approach middle age and beyond, they wonder about what affect their hypothyroidism will have on them in future years. Others, who are diagnosed in their fifties, sixties, and older, also wonder about becoming hypothyroid and what that means for them as they age.

There are many factors regarding how we age that are out of our control. Genetics, childhood development, and past health practices are all things that we can't do anything about now (at least, not yet). But we can control a great deal from this day forward, and everything we do to promote our health and well-being will have a great impact on the extent of our health picture for years to come.

Diet, exercise, and range of motion

A good, balanced diet combined with a regular exercise program that promotes stamina, stretching, and strength will enable your body to fuel its activity and maintain a foundation of good habits now and in the future. Letting go of deleterious habits, such as smoking, taking illegal drugs, or drinking inappropriate amounts of alcohol will also pay you great dividends in the future. As you age, allowing for your body's changes and modifying your exercise and eating habits will also help you reduce the stress to your joints while still doing things that help you.

Keeping medically current

I was amazed when, at a recent American Thyroid Association conference, a physician said the greatest impediment to getting good results from treating hypothyroid patients with medication was that of patient compliance. One study indicated that of the 365 days of prescribed medication, the average patient only takes 265 days' worth of meds! This means that many patients aren't getting the thyroid hormone that they should—and it's no wonder that some patients don't feel markedly better once they start thyroid medication!

You can help your healthful future by being consistent now with taking your medication, as well as monitoring your health and keeping your doctor's and lab appointments current. No one can make you take your medication except you, and although it isn't great to have to take pills, the alternative is that your body will not have enough thyroid hormone to function optimally . . . and you won't feel as well as you could. Of course, if you are taking your meds and still don't feel relief, you should explore alternatives and/or possibly other diagnoses with your doctor. But you should also take the thyroid medication as and when prescribed by your doctor so that he or she (and you) can truly know if it is helping.

"Premature" aging

One of the signs of increased risk for a thyroid problem is prematurely gray hair (defined as "one gray hair before thirty").[1] As minute as this detail might seem, it does help illustrate the close connection between some signs of what we would usually consider "just aging" and the effects of low thyroid function.

Other symptoms of hypothyroidism might also be misconstrued as "just aging": fatigue, weight gain, forgetfulness, dry skin or hair, hair loss, and menstrual irregularities. But as you now know, because the thyroid gland's hormones regulate so many bodily functions, it is no wonder that, as we slow down due to hypothyroidism, we *feel* as though we are getting older.

If left untreated, hypothyroidism can progress to something very debilitating. In the most extreme cases, it can lead to a kind of dementia very similar to that experienced by Alzheimer's patients. But if you are reading this book, you know that there is help for hypothyroidism. If you get the appropriate medical care and pay close attention to other areas of your health and life, you should be able to feel relief in your hypothyroid symptoms and, eventually, feel younger than you have since before you started treatment.

Looking inside out

Many older people say that if they keep their mind active, they feel younger than their calendar years. If you haven't already done so, now is the time to find a good way to manage stress and keep your intellectual, spiritual, and emotional life vibrant and whole. Learning how to be proactive in difficult situations and practicing "diplomatic assertiveness" to stand up for yourself will protect your future health tremendously and give you a fine sense of self-esteem and self-worth. Learning a new subject, taking up a new hobby, or just opening your mind and heart to the myriad of possibilities for new information around you can help you achieve a youth that transcends your age.

A support group of friends and loved ones can be wonderful for your healthful future, but just as important is making sure you are a friend and loved one to them. Look inside yourself to see where you can be better at building quality, nurturing relationships. Find the wonderful parts of your spirit and personality that you can share with others and feel the joy of being able to give back without expecting in return.

IN A SENTENCE:

Although there are some things that are out of our control, being healthy in the future means developing and embracing healthful habits now.

learning

Aging and Hypothyroidism

ACCORDING TO the Thyroid Foundation of America, by age fifty, 10 percent of women have signs of thyroid failure. By age sixty, this percentage goes up to 17 percent of women and 8 percent of men.[2] It is no wonder, then, that the TFA recommends TSH testing for anyone over the age of fifty or who has symptoms.[3]

But you already have hypothyroidism and you know the importance of having your thyroid levels monitored at least once a year after your levels and medication have stabilized. Is there anything else you should be watching out for? Do you have a predisposition to developing any other illness or auto-immune disease?

Vital organs

If you have been hyperthyroid in the past, or if your hypothyroidism has been severe, you should have your heart checked by a competent cardiologist to make sure there is no damage stemming from your thyroid disease. Also, you should have your cholesterol levels checked, especially if your thyroid disease is still fluctuating as your gland burns out.

Usually, hypothyroidism does not have lasting effects on your other organs. Still, you should have regular checkups to make sure that your organs are functioning well and that you aren't lacking in any nutrients.

If you have been treated for hyperthyroidism, or are on high doses of thyroid hormone, you should also have a bone density test. This painless, quick procedure will be able to indicate if you are losing bone mass and thus could be at risk for osteoporosis. There are many treatments for osteoporosis now, including taking calcium supplements and/or prescription drugs; as long as you catch the problem before it is too severe, you should be able to treat it successfully.

One thing I noticed about treating my hypothyroidism was that my asthma got considerably better. My allergist told me that there is a correlation between hypothyroidism and aggravated asthma, and that treating the thyroid problem can sometimes improve the breathing problems. This has certainly happened in my case; you might want to speak about this relationship with your doctor if you suffer from asthma.

Menopause

Menopause is the process through which a woman's ovaries stop functioning. It includes hormonal changes that signal the end of a woman's ability to ovulate and ends with the absence of menstruation. As with the symptoms of premature aging, some hypothyroid patients feel as though they are going through early menopause. Their symptoms are certainly similar: "hot flashes," irregular menstrual periods, irritability, dry skin/hair/vagina, and hair loss.

There could be some thyroid-related reasons for early menopause. For example, chemotherapy and radiation treatment of thyroid cancer can bring about early menopause, as can extreme hypothyroidism that affects the pituitary gland's function and, thus, the menstruation-inducing hormone process. But often the "menopause" symptoms a hypothyroid woman feels are due to the thyroid condition itself and they clear up once the hormone levels are brought back into the normal range, especially if the woman is younger than forty-five years old. (Usually, menopause occurs between the ages of forty-five and fifty-two.)

There are many hormonal tests that a gynecologist or endocrinologist can run that can help decipher the mystery of what's going on inside your body besides hypothyroidism. Before you explore alternative therapies or herbs for your symptoms, seek medical assistance from one of these specialists and see what they have to say.

Hormone Replacement Therapy (HRT)

Menopause is a very natural part of aging, and many women choose to ride it out, carefully keeping in mind potential problems, such as osteoporosis, that might ensue at the end of it. Other women, hypothyroid and "healthy," have chosen to take hormone replacement therapy (HRT) to a greater or lesser degree. In recent months, this treatment has become quite controversial because of some scientific information that indicates it might increase the risk of some cancers.

The best thing I can tell you about HRT is that you should keep close to your doctor as information is sorted out about the short- and long-term effects on otherwise healthy, as well as chronically ill women. Monitor some of the Web sites listed in the Resources section, too, to get current information. And don't feel "out of step" if you choose to go through menopause naturally. Many women have done so before you and lived to quite active, old ages!

The course of the hypo-active thyroid gland

If you have Hashimoto's thyroiditis, you know that your thyroid hormone levels can fluctuate, sometimes wildly. In fact, you might have periods when you are hypo- then hyperthyroid and return to being hypothyroid. Such is the unpredictable course of the disease. But somewhere along the line, your gland will "burn itself out," and you will need to be on a full (for you) course of thyroid replacement for the rest of your life.

There is usually no health complication or side effect to having full replacement therapy. Unless you develop a large goiter or thyroid cancer, you should not have to have your inactive gland removed. As long as you keep monitoring your condition and seeking appropriate medical attention, you should be able to look forward to a full and productive life.

IN A SENTENCE:

> *In Hashimoto's thyroiditis, the thyroid gland eventually "burns itself out," but the health effects from this and taking lifelong thyroid supplement are usually not damaging to your overall health.*

Who Cares?

BY NOW, you are seeing your doctor less frequently than you had when you first started treatment, and you are also getting your thyroid checked at longer intervals. You are more on your own to juggle the many demands of having a chronic illness and living your full life, and you might find yourself wondering if there's anything going on in the great world "out there" regarding new treatments, diagnostic procedures, or cures for hypothyroidism.

"Who cares?" you might ask.

The answer is: A lot of people.

The "big" picture

Thyroid disease is not just an illness, it is a public health issue. Each year, millions of people experience a dip in their productivity, rising medical costs, and other disruptions to their lives because they are hypothyroid (or hyperthyroid). Other people are thrust into a world of cancer surgery and treatment when they find out that their thyroid gland has nodules that have become cancerous or the cancer has metastasized (spread beyond the thyroid gland), and they and their loved ones suddenly find themselves engaged in a lifelong fight. Still other people don't know that they are hypothyroid, but they *feel* awful; even if they are not diagnosed, they still have the symptoms and, thus, the effects upon their work and outside lives that others do.

The toll that thyroid disease takes on the public productivity, economy, and overall health is enormous. Thankfully, the American Thyroid Association (ATA) has been promoting awareness and research since 1923, and the National Institutes of Health has long funded thyroid research. NIH research levels are not what everyone would wish, and future attention to and funding for thyroid research is not necessarily expected to grow. However, there are some things that are happening that are aimed at raising more awareness and protecting the public, at least in some specific areas.

Terrorism and the thyroid

Unfortunately, we now live in a country that is vulnerable to attack from people who seek to destroy us. One of the current threats to our way of life is potential terrorist attacks on our country's nuclear power plants. Such catastrophes could have far-reaching consequences to the survivors' health, sense of security, and quality of life.

As was seen in Chernobyl in the former Soviet Union, nuclear radiation can severely affect the health of the thyroid gland. Several thousand people who as children were in the path of the radioactive fallout from the Chernobyl plant's meltdown have developed thyroid nodules or an unusually aggressive form of thyroid cancer. The U.S. Food and Drug Administration (FDA) has approved over-the-counter potassium iodide pills that are available at some pharmacies and through the Internet. The U.S. Nuclear Regulatory Commission (NRC) gives these pills to states that request them, to protect people living within certain distances of nuclear power plants.

As of the end of 2002, the planned Department of Homeland Security may take over potassium iodide stockpiling and distribution as part of the overall response to nuclear threats. In the event of a plant failure or a terrorist attack, people would be advised to take the potassium iodide to protect their thyroid gland from damage due to uptake of concentrated levels of radioactive iodine released by the explosion. As with Chernobyl, the need for potassium iodide is greatest for babies and children. (People who have had their thyroid gland removed don't need potassium iodide, as there is usually minimal to no thyroid tissue left to absorb the radioactive iodine.)

You can learn more about potassium iodide at Web sites for the FDA (http://www.fda.gov/cder/drugprepare/KI_Q&A.htm), NRC (http://www. nrc.gov/what-we-do/regulatory/emer-resp/emer-prep/ki-faq.html), and the American Thyroid Association (www.thyroid.org) and in the patient materials that it distributes. Your doctor should also be up to date on your need for and the availability of potassium iodide. If you live near a nuclear power plant, be sure you discuss the issue of potassium iodide with your doctor and keep informed about developments regarding protecting you, your family, and your health.

Thyroid Awareness Month

January is Thyroid Awareness Month. Endocrinologists and other thyroid specialists are particularly attuned to spreading the word about the thyroid gland and its functions during this time—and you can be, too. Here's how:

○ In advance of January, obtain information from the American Thyroid Association, Thyroid Foundation of America, Thyroid Foundation of Canada, National Graves' Disease Foundation, ThyCA: Thyroid Cancer Survivors' Association, or Light of Life Foundation (for patients with thyroid cancer), and distribute it to family and friends.

○ Contact the local media (newspapers, radio, and television stations) and ask them to do stories on what thyroid disease is and what to do about it.

○ See if any hospitals or universities in your area are hosting health fairs and ask to participate in them, or encourage them to provide thyroid screening tests to the people who attend.

○ In conjunction with the local chapter of your chosen thyroid focused organization, put together a daylong symposium for thyroid patients and their loved ones. Include talks by doctors and mental health professionals and testimonials from patients to make the event as well rounded as possible.

You might think that your individual efforts to get the word out about thyroid disease will be too small to be noticed. Unlike with other diseases and causes, thyroid disease *is* woefully underrepresented in national advertisements, commercials, and public service announcements. But your becoming involved at the local level in raising awareness *will* contribute to the national cause and make a huge difference in many people's lives. Starting from the "grass roots" and building from there is a very good place to begin.

Researchers

Medical research on thyroid function and treatments for thyroid disease is ongoing in many places throughout the world. In the U.S., such work happens in university and hospital research departments, the National Institutes of Health (NIH) and other governmental agencies, and pharmaceutical companies' laboratories.

Researchers come from a variety of backgrounds; some are medical doctors (M.D.s), while others have specific training in areas of biology and organic chemistry relating to endocrinology and thyroid function. Typically, these workers don't make a lot of money; their love of investigation and discovery is what drives them to withstand the long hours, dead ends, and tedious process of scientific research. Their monetary support comes from several sources, including government and institutional research grants, foundation donations, and pharmaceutical company funding. Individuals can help, too, by contributing in any amount (even small contributions make a *big* difference) to specific research projects or foundations and organizations.

Future activities

Should everyone be tested for thyroid disease?

The Thyroid Foundation of America estimates that approximately eight million Americans have hypothyroidism and don't know it.[1] Whether this is due to Hashimoto's thyroiditis or other thyroid function failure is unknown. But current statistics bear out that there are many people who might need supplemental thyroid hormone, but aren't even aware that they have a medical problem.

Whether there will be nationwide thyroid screening to identify and eventually treat these people is unclear at present. But the dialogue has begun. Your involvement in raising awareness about thyroid disease can help promote nationwide screening and move more people to get help for their seemingly baffling symptoms.

IN A SENTENCE:

> *Increasing awareness of thyroid problems will help the millions of patients with untreated thyroid disease to get an accurate diagnosis and treatment.*

learning

The Latest in Research and Treatments

THERE IS no cure for hypothyroidism and, because it can be treated effectively, there are really no plans to find one (there is little to no financial incentive for the drug companies to develop one). However there is a lot of research going on all over the world concerning thyroid function, levels of "normal," pre-, during-, and post-natal care of mother and child, as well as other issues relating to autoimmunity in general and specifically to thyroid disease.

Causes of thyroid disease

One of the areas that scientists are now focusing on is that of the genetic and environmental triggers to developing thyroid disease and, specifically, hypothyroidism. Previous and ongoing studies include looking at stress, cigarette smoke, and the relationship between autoimmune thyroid disease and other autoimmune illnesses in some patients, as well as family history and thyroid disease (or other autoimmune disease development).

Subclinical hypothyroidism

This controversial area of hypothyroidism was of particular interest at the seventy-fourth annual meeting of the American

Thyroid Association (ATA). Subclinical hypothyroidism is considered present when a patient has a high TSH but a normal or almost normal T_4. The presence of symptoms in subclinical hypothyroid patients varies, and some doctors hesitate to give thyroid hormone to them. One study presented at the ATA meeting concluded that "subjects with SCHypo (subclinical hypothyroidism) have subtle decrements in quality of life."[2] But further study is needed before there is a consensus among treating physicians about whether people with subclinical hypothyroidism should take thyroid hormone therapy.

Effects of hypothyroidism on internal organs

To date, there have been some, but not nearly enough, studies about the long-term effects of hypothyroidism on the heart, lungs, brain, and other internal organs. One reason for this is that thyroid patients (and many other people) are living longer than ever before, and so have more time to develop hypothyroid-related problems. Hypothyroidism and its effects on the unborn, as well as newborn, child are being well documented, but there is still a large gap in the literature as it concerns adults.

T_4, T_3, or both?

Anecdotally, some hypothyroid patients say that they feel better on a combination of T_4 and T_3, while others say they don't notice much of a difference. Some physicians say that many of their patients feel better on a combination of the two hormones for about a month, and then end up feeling worse. In my own experience, I haven't noticed a marked difference. Thyroidologists are actively looking at the short- and long-term benefits and drawbacks of combination therapy for hypothyroidism. It might be frustrating to have to wait for a while, but I'm confident that in the future, perhaps not long from now, we will have some scientifically based answers to this controversial question.

Hypothyroidism and pregnancy

This is an especially important area of research because of the long-term impact hypothyroidism can have on both the mother and child. Thyroidologists often team up with reproductive endocrinologists to study areas such as fetal brain development, genetic propensity to develop auto-immune illness, and post-natal cognitive follow-up.

Getting involved in what we still need to know

I've presented the areas where we still need more research to give you a sense of the "work in progress" of thyroidology. Now, is there anything you can do about it?

One thing you can do is consider being part of a clinical trial or other study.

Throughout the country, in universities and labs, hospitals and phar-maceutical companies, studies are being conducted on these and other issues concerning hypothyroidism. Your doctor probably knows of studies being conducted, especially in your area. Also, lists of clinical trials and studies are posted on Web sites, such as the NIH's site (www.nih.gov), and through other medical associations, such as the American Association of Clinical Endocrinologists (AACE).

Usually, the parameters of the study are listed (what issue is being stud-ied and what type of people/symptoms/illness is/are to be included in the study population), as well as the duration of the study and a contact per-son and their telephone number and address. Sometimes, patients involved in studies are compensated for their time and/or expenses. Rarely do they have to pay for anything connected with the study.

If you find a study that you think you might be appropriate for, contact the person organizing it and ask the following questions:

○ What information do you need from me (tests, family history, etc.) before deciding if I can participate?
○ What is expected of me during the study (time involved, travel [if any]), compliance with taking medication)?
○ What, if any, expenses will I incur as a result of the study? For what will I be reimbursed?
○ Are there any potential side effects or other dangers to participat-ing in the study?
○ Will I be able to leave the study before it is completed if I no longer want to be a part of it?

○ Will there be any long-term follow-up (do I need to continue to be available weeks, months, or years from now)?

Speak with your doctor before agreeing to participate in a study, especially if you have health issues besides hypothyroidism. Also talk with your family, particularly if the study requires their participation or if it will take you away from them for any period of time.

If you decide to participate in a study, you should feel very good about it. You will be making a very important contribution to the health of many people, including yourself.

Why does it take so long to get answers?

Before they are able to begin, researchers must go through elaborate processes to plan, find funding for, and apply for permission and funding to conduct their studies. Clinical trials and studies might go on for months or years before scientists are able to come to any conclusions concerning a cause or treatment for an illness. New drugs, too, have to go through a painstaking process of development, trial, error, and approval before they can be brought to market.

In today's fast-paced world, it is often easy to become frustrated with the seemingly slow pace of modern science and to turn to more anecdotally based data and therapeutic "fixes" because of that impatience. But in the long run, taking time to find reasons and appropriate treatments for hypothyroidism will hold doctors and patients in good stead. More will be understood about potential side effects, dosages, and pathologies of illness. And less will be left up to the opinion of people who don't have the background or experience in the art and science of medicine.

IN A SENTENCE:

> There's still so much to learn about hypothyroidism and there are many clinical trials and studies conducted throughout the country to help answer these questions and solve these mysteries.

living

You've Come a Long Way!

A WHOLE year has gone by! Can you believe it?

And in this first year, you have taken your health condition firmly by the roots and cultivated a healthier, stronger, more resilient you. You have gained invaluable insight about how your body works and how you can enable yourself to maintain control over your health and any problems that might occur. You have a support system of friends, family, and medical professionals who are dedicated to helping you. And you have come through a year of trial with beautiful, flying colors!

All of this and more is cause for joy, hope, great faith, and celebration. You should feel good about yourself in a way that you never have, and proud of all that you've accomplished. Even though you know that you will be living with hypothyroidism for the rest of your life, you know that the days, weeks, and years to come need not only be devoted to keeping your head above water. Rather, you can be hypothyroid and still SOAR!

The implications of all you've been through this year and all that you have accomplished might seem clearly evident now. But you will find, as you continue into the next year and beyond, that the foundation you've laid for yourself will continue to surprise, delight, and inspire you. Your newly honed health habits will accompany you through childbirth, raising children, excelling at your chosen profession, and aging gracefully and with a sense of contentment and peace that others might envy.

Just as important as how you've triumphed are the skills you've acquired to help you through the challenges that might lie ahead. You know what to do if you feel depressed, if you suspect that your thyroid hormones might not be sufficient, and if you are dissatisfied with your healthcare, medical team, or medication. You know your body well enough to be able to tell your doctor what hurts, what's "off," and give him or her enough quantifiable information to help reach a correct diagnosis. You know how to cope with pain, disappointment, fatigue, and sorrow. And you know it's all right to cry and be angry—and how to keep this from preventing you from living in an overall healthy manner.

The dreams and goals you had before your diagnosis might have to be modified a bit now that you have a chronic illness. But that doesn't mean you have to set them aside. Throughout this past year, you've learned how to be realistic about setting priorities and balancing your health needs with the desires of your heart. Perhaps your dreams and goals have changed in light of this insight. But whatever you want to do in the future, you are confident that hypothyroidism need not deter you. If anything, it will spur you on to be more of a dreamer, and more of an achiever. Indeed, feeling your *worst* can bring out the *best* in you and turn your life into a marvel that holds never-ending good surprises and achievements.

IN A SENTENCE:

At the end of this first year, you are a stronger person, filled with growing wisdom about your body, your heart, and your soul.

learning

What You Can Do to Celebrate

THERE IS nothing better than triumphing over adversity. And, now that you've lived through your first year with hypothyroidism, you *know* adversity. You've experienced pain, loss, deep sorrow, and harsh physical symptoms. But more importantly, you've not just survived, you've thrived! And you've faced the challenges of one short year with courage, strength, humor, and resilience. Think of all you've been through, all you've learned, and all you've become. You should feel a sense of accomplishment and gratitude for overcoming these extreme obstacles. You should also feel stronger for being tested in the fire of illness and more empathetic toward others who are going through similar trials.

It is this empathy that might fuel in you a deep determination to help others, to give them some of the knowledge and encouragement that helped you get through your "dark night of the soul." After all, in small and significant ways, others helped you to survive and grow. In fact, many of these people are still a presence in your life, encouraging you, heartening you, and rejoicing with you in your triumphs. Giving back to others is an excellent way to celebrate your newfound wholeness, and it is more than good to follow through with this feeling—it is wonderful!

One way that you can "give back" is to step up your involvement in one or more of the patient support groups that helped you through this year. You might want to become a support leader, or you might want to participate in a clinical trial. Monetary contributions are always welcome by nonprofit organizations, but so are volunteer hours. If you don't think you can give a lot of time in patient support, perhaps you can offer to help with mailings, Web site maintenance, or other forms of volunteering.

If there is a hospital near you, you might offer to volunteer there, working with patients who are admitted for thyroid-related reasons (thyroid cancer patients, perhaps). Your firsthand understanding and empathy will make a tremendous difference in their lives. On a personal level, you will undoubtedly hear of a friend, or a friend of a friend, who has developed hypothyroidism and is struggling with fatigue, depression, and other symptoms. Reaching out to him or her is another excellent way of moving forward with your own condition (you'll realize even more fully how far you've come) and you'll be making a difference in someone else's life as well.

Beyond specifically working with other hypothyroid patients, medical professionals, or the organizations that offer support and information to them, you might want to explore a whole new avenue of employment that includes counseling, teaching, healthcare work, or another service-oriented profession. It is all right to change careers, especially if you have been so deeply moved by your own experience. In fact, there is nothing worse than being in an "ill-fitting" job where you can't make full use of your talents and skills. You have unlimited potential if you are working in a field and in an occupation that is "just right."

Keep learning

As you've seen, there are still many areas of thyroidology that need to be identified and explored. Because this world of healthcare is constantly evolving, it is important for you to keep learning about your condition, to build on what you already know and increase your perspective on what lies ahead. Many of the organizations and sources of continuing knowledge can be found in the Resources section. You can use them as a springboard and continue adding to your knowledge—and share what you learn with others who are also living with hypothyroidism.

In health and happiness

As you approach your next year with hypothyroidism and beyond, know that you will still have to monitor your health and take care of your condition, as well as your overall health picture. There will still be stresses that buffet you, challenges that you will need to face. But there won't be another "First Year" like the one you just had! There will only be years when you can build upon what you've learned, forge ahead to new productivity, growth, and joy. And move on to each day with renewed happiness.

For, you did it! You made it through!

And now, the rest is up to you.

IN A SENTENCE:

> *During this first year, you have acquired invaluable knowledge and insight about yourself and your hypothyroidism, and you are ready to continue learning and living to your fullest health potential and realizing your deepest personal dreams.*

BALLARD STREET Jerry Van Amerongen

Linda's new pills are a godsend.

By permission of Jerry Van Amerongen and Creators Syndicate, Inc.

Glossary

Note: The definitions given here are written to correspond to the text of this book and hypothyroidism; they are not meant to be complete medical definitions.

ALOPECIA AREATA: Hair loss in one area of the head.

ALOPECIA TOTALIS: Loss of all the hair on one's head.

ALOPECIA UNIVERSALIS: Loss of all scalp and body hair (except sometimes the pubic hair).

ANABOLIC: The phase of the metabolic process where cells are "built up."

ANDROGENETIC ALOPECIA: Hereditary pattern baldness that can affect men and women.

ANTIBODY: In a healthy person, antibodies (immunoglobulin molecules) are part of the immune system that protects the body from "invaders," i.e., diseases, allergens. In autoimmune diseases, the antibodies turn against the body's own tissues and organs, attacking them as if they were the "invaders."

APOPROTEIN: A protein that carries fat (cholesterol) throughout the body via the blood.

ARRHYTHMIA: Irregular, especially of heartbeats.

AUTOIMMUNE: Immunity against one's own tissues or organs.

BODY MASS INDEX (BMI): The measure of body fat percentage based on height and weight and provides four categories: Underweight, Normal Weight, Overweight, Obesity. Applies to adult men and women.

CATABOLIC: The phase of the metabolic process where energy is released as "fuel" for the body's cells.

CHOLESTEROL: A lipid (fat) that circulates throughout the body, affecting the structure and function of all your cells and also having a part in the formation of hormones.

CRETENISM: Underdevelopment of a child's physio-psychological systems.

ENDOCRINE: Of or pertaining to internal glands that secrete hormones that affect various organs and systems within the body.

ENDOCRINOLOGIST: A medical doctor with extra training in and a professional designation to treat and/or research diseases and syndromes pertaining to the endocrine (hormonal) system.

EUTHYROID: A condition where the patient has normal TSH and normal T_4.

GOITROGEN: A chemical found in some foods that interferes with the thyroid gland's ability to produce hormone.

HAIR FOLLICLE: A tiny organ on the head or elsewhere on the body from which a single hair grows.

HEMOTOLOGIST: A medical professional who specializes in disorders and tests of the blood.

HIGH-DENSITY LIPOPROTEIN (HDL): The "good" cholesterol, which prevents buildup of plaque in the arteries.

HORMONE: A glandular secretion that travels through the internal system of blood passageways to the body's organs and which affects these organs' functions.

HYPEROCHOLESTEROLEMIA: High cholesterol.

HYPERTHYROIDISM: A condition where the thyroid gland produces too much metabolic hormone.

HYPOTHYROIDISM: A condition where the thyroid gland produces too little metabolic hormone.

HYPOTHALAMUS: The gland that secretes thyroid releasing hormone (TRH) to the pituitary.

IODIDE: A component of iodine and essential to the production of adequate levels of T_4 and the conversion of T_4 to T_3.

IODINE: An element, present in salt and other food substances that is absorbed by the thyroid gland and used in the production of thyroid hormone.

LIPOPROTEIN: A combination of a fat (lipid) and a protein that carries the lipid throughout the bloodstream.

LOW-DENSITY LIPOPROTEIN (LDL): The "bad" cholesterol, which causes buildup of cholesterol in the arteries.

METABOLIC RATE: The pace at which your metabolism functions.

METABOLISM: The intricate physical and chemical system by which your body develops, grows, and functions.

NATURAL [MEDICATION]: A product derived from organic substances, such as plant or animal tissue.

ONCOLOGIST: A medical doctor (M.D.) who specializes in treating cancer.

OPHTHALMOLOGIST: A medical doctor (M.D.) who treats disorders and diseases of the eye.

OSTEOPOROSIS: A condition in which bones lose their substance, or "mass," and become brittle to the point of disintegrating and breaking.

PITUITARY: A gland located at the base of the brain that secretes hormone affecting various body functions, including the production of thyroid stimulating hormone (TSH).

SELECTIVE SEROTONIN REUPTAKE INHIBITOR (SSRI): Antidepressant that increases the amount of serotonin in your brain. Used to treat some forms of depression.

SEROTONIN: A chemical produced by the brain that helps to regulate mood.

SUBCLINICAL HYPOTHYROIDISM: So-defined in patients with normal or almost normal T_4, high TSH, and some or no symptoms of hypothyroidism.

SYNTHETIC [MEDICATION]: A product with the same chemical characteristics as a natural [medication] product, but which is produced using non-organic substances.

T LYMPHOCYTE: A type of white blood cell involved in the immune process.

TETRACYCLIC ANTIDEPRESSANT: Medication used to treat depression that affects neurotransmitters by a different mechanism than SSRIs.

THYROIDOLOGIST: Someone (usually a physician or researcher with a Ph.D.) who devotes his or her research and work to the study of various aspects of the thyroid.

THYROIDOLOGY: The study of disorders and pathologies related to the thyroid gland and its function.

TRICYCLIC ANTIDEPRESSANT: Medication used to treat depression that affects neurotransmitters by a different mechanism than SSRIs.

Notes

Introduction

1. Mayo Clinic statistics of prevalence and demographics—http://www.mayoclinic.com/findinformation/diseaseandconditions/invoke.cfm?id=DS00353.

Day 1

1. Lawrence Woods, M.D. "The Most Common Problem—Hypo-thyroidism." Thyroid Foundation of America. http://66.129.68.207/disorders/hypothyroidism.
2. "Facts about Thyroid Cancer," ThyCA: Thyroid Cancer Survivors' Association, Inc. www.thyca.org.
3. Nobuyuki Amino, M.D. (revised). "Hashimoto's Thyroiditis," The Thyroid and Its Diseases. http://www.thyroidmanager.org/Chapter8/8-text.htm.
4. "Questions and Answers about Potassium Iodide (KI)," Press release from the American Thyroid Association, September 28, 2002. Available at www.thyroid.org.

Day 2

1. "AACE Clinical Practice Guidelines for the Evaluation and Treatment of Hyperthyroidism and Hypothyroidism." Developed by the American Association of Clinical Endocrinologists and the American College of Endocrinology. 1994.

2. "Subclinical Hypothyroidism During Pregnancy: Position Statement from the American Association of Clinical Endocrinologists." Gharib, Cobin, and Dickey. 1999.
3. Ibid.

Day 3

1. Lawrence Woods, M.D. "The Most Common Problem – Hypothyroidism." Thyroid Foundation of America. http://66.129.68.207/disorders/hypothyroidism.
2. *Companion Encyclopedia of the History of Medicine, Volume One*. W. F. Bynum and Roy Porter, editors. Routledge. London & New York. 1993. Pages 498–499. Material also from personal interview with Basil Rapoport, M.B., thyroidologist. Los Angeles. 2002.
3. Gilbert H. Daniels, M.D. "Getting Practical: How to Treat Patients with Thyroid Hypofunction." American Thyroid Association Annual Meeting. Los Angeles, 2002.

Day 4

1. "Hair Loss." Patient information from the American Academy of Dermatology Web site. http://www.aad.org/pamphlets/hairloss.html.

Day 6

1. "Diagnosing Depression," Mayoclinic.com. http://www.mayoclinic.com/findinformation/conditioncenters/invoke.cfm?objectid=916C.
2. "AACE Clinical Practice Guidelines for the Evaluation and Treatment of Hyperthyroidism and Hypothyroidism." Developed by the American Association of Clinical Endocrinologists and the American College of Endocrinology. 1994
3. Larry Dossey, M.D. *Healing Words: The Power of Prayer and the Practice of Medicine*. Harperpaperbacks. 1997.
4. Harold G. Koenig, M.D. *The Healing Power of Faith*. Simon and Schuster. 1999.

Day 7

1. "A Collaborative Study of the Genetics of Anorexia Nervosa and Bulimia Nervosa." Chief investigator Walter H. Kaye, M.D., University of Pittsburgh, Pittsburgh, PA. http://www.wpic.pitt.edu/research/pranbn/index.html.
2. "'Miracle' Health Claims: Add a Dose of Skepticism," Federal Trade Commission in cooperation with the Food and Drug Administration. http://www.ftc.gov/bcp/conline/pubs/health/frdheal.htm.
3. "Dietary Guidelines: Choose Sensibly." http://www.health.gov/dietaryguidelines/dga2000/document/choose.htm.

Week 3

1. Nobuyuki Amino, M.D. (revised). "Hashimoto's Thyroiditis," The Thyroid and Its Diseases. http://www.thyroidmanager.org/Chapter8/8-text.htm.

2. Daniel J. Wallace, M.D. *The Lupus Book*. Revised and expanded edition. Oxford University Press, 2000. Page 13.
3. "Autoimmune Thyroid Diseases," from *Thyroid Signpost*, Volume 1, Number 5. Patient information provided by the Thyroid Society for Education and Research. 1993, 1996.

Week 4

1. "Frequently Asked Questions and Answers," U.S. Department of Labor. Elaws – FMLA Advisor. http://www.elaws.dol.gov/fmla/wren/faq.htm.
2. "ADA at a glance," iCanonline. http://www.icanonline.net. ALSO: www. disAbility.gov

Month 7

1. Daniel Glinoer, M.D., Ph.D., "Keynote Clinical Address: Thyroid Disease in Pregnancy," 74th Annual meeting of the American Thyroid Association. Los Angeles, 2002.
2. Ibid.
3. "Subclinical Hypothyroidism During Pregnancy: Position Statement from the American Association of Clinical Endorinologists." Gharib, Cobin, and Dickey. 1999.

Month 10

1. "Do you have a thyroid risk?" Patient education information supplied by Thyroid Foundation of America. www.allthyroid.org.
2. Elliot G.Levy, M.D. "Thyroid Problems over 50." Thyroid Foundation of America. http://66.129.68.207/disorders/aging/over50.
3. Ibid.

Month 11

1. Lawrence C. Wood, M.D. "The Most Common Problem—Hypothyroidism." Patient information provided by the Thyroid Foundation of America. http:// 66.129.68.207/disorders/hypothyroidism.
2. "Effects of Experimentally Induced Subclinical Hypothyroidism on Quality of Life and Mood," Samuels, M., Schuff, K., Carello, P., Janowsky, J. Oregon Health and Science University, Portland, Oregon, USA. Poster presented at 74th annual meeting of the American Thyroid Society. October 2002.

For Further Reading

Dossey, Larry, M.D. *Healing Words: The Power of Prayer and the Practice of Medicine*. HarperPaperbacks, 1993.

Greenberg, Peter. *The Travel Detective*. Villard, 2001.

_____. *Flight Crew Confidential*. Villard, 2002.

Koenig, Harold G., M.D. *The Healing Power of Faith*. Simon and Schuster, 1999.

Marek, Claudia Craig. *The First Year™—Fibromyalgia*. Marlowe & Co., 2002.

Pratt, Maureen, and David Hallegua, M.D. *Taking Charge of Lupus: How to Manage the Disease and Make the Most of Your Life*. New American Library, 2002.

Rosenthal, M. Sara. *The Thyroid Sourcebook, 3rd Edition*. Lowell House, 1998.

_____. *The Thyroid Sourcebook for Women*. Lowell House, 1999.

Wallace, Daniel J., and Janice Brock Wallace. *Making Sense of Fibromyalgia*. Oxford University Press, 2000.

Resources

Note: Much of today's information, especially up-to-the-minute news, is best accessed on the Internet. This is terrific for people who have home computers or have access to one at work or through friends, but might seem out of reach for those who don't.

If you do not have or cannot afford a computer and Internet access, you can still benefit from the World Wide Web. Many public libraries offer computers free of charge (although they might limit the amount of time you spend "surfing"). Your doctor's office might agree to let you use the computer there, if you can't afford to purchase one yourself. Also, your college alumni association, church or synagogue, and/or other civic organization might have a computer that you can use.

Organizations

The American Association of Clinical Endocrinologists
2589 Park Street
Jacksonville, FL 32204-4554
Telephone: 904-384-9490
Fax: 904-384-8124
Web: www.aace.org
Web site devoted to thyroid:
  www.thyroidmanager.org

American Chiropractic Association
1701 Clarendon Blvd.
Arlington, VA 22209
Telephone (toll-free): 1-800-986-4636
Fax: 703-243-2593
Web: www.amerchiro.org

American Foundation of Thyroid Patients
P.O. Box 820195
Houston, TX 77282-0195
Toll-free telephone: 888-006-4460
Telephone: 281-496-4460
Fax: 281-496-0369
Web: www.thyroidfoundation.org

The American Thyroid Association
6066 Leesburg Pike, Suite 650
Falls Church, VA 22041
Telephone: 703-998-8890
Fax: 703-998-8893
Email: admin@thyroid.org
Web: www.thyroid.org

The Arthritis Foundation
P.O. Box 7669
Atlanta, GA 30357-0669
Telephone (toll-free): 1-800-207-8633
Arthritis Answers (toll-free):
  1-800-283-7800
Web: www.arthritis.org

The Endocrine Society
4350 East West Highway
Suite 500
Bethesda, MD 20814
Telephone: 310-941-0200
Fax: 301-941-0259
Email: endostaff@endo-society.org
Web: www.endo-society.org

Magic Foundation (support and education for families of children with growth disorders)
1327 N. Harlem Avenue
Oak Park, IL 60302
Phone: 708-383-0808
Fax: 708-383-0899
Web: www.magicfoundation.org

MedicAlert Foundation
2323 Colorado Avenue
Turlock, CA 95382
Telephone for membership (toll-free):
  1-800-863-3420
Web: www.medicalert.org

National Alopecia Areata Foundation
P.O. Box 150760
San Rafael, CA 94915-0760
Phone: 415-456-4644
Fax: 415-456-4274
Email: info@naaf.ort
Web: www.naaf.org

National Graves' Disease Foundation
P.O. Box 1969
Brevard, NC 28712
Phone: 828-877-5251
Fax: 828-877-5250
Email: ngdf@citcom.nct
Web: www.ngdf.org

ThyCa: Thyroid Cancer Survivors' Association, Inc.
P.O. Box 1545
New York, NY 10159-1545
Phone (toll-free): 1-877-588-7904
Fax: 630-604-6078
Email: thyca@thyca.org
Web: www.thyca.org

Thyroid Foundation of America, Inc.
410 Stuart Street
Boston, MA 02116
Phone (toll free): 1-800-832-8321
Phone: 617-534-1500
Fax: 617-534-1515
Email: info@allthyroid.org
Web: www.allthyroid.org

Thyroid Foundation of Canada
P.O. Box/CP 1919 Stn Main
Kingston, Ontario K7L537
Phone: 613-544-8364
Fax: 613-544-9731
Web: www.thyroid.ca

"tlc" (The American Cancer Society's company that carries fashionable hats and other head coverings for women experiencing hair loss)
340 Poplar Street
Hanover, PA 17333-0080
Telephone (toll-free): 1-800-850-9445
Fax (toll-free): 1-800-757-9997
Web: www.tlccatalog.org

U.S. Department of Justice Civil Rights Division
(Information about Americans with Disabilities Act)
P.O. Box 66118
Washington, DC 20035-6118
Telephone (toll-free): 1-800-514-0301
TDD (toll-free): 1-800-514-0383

Pharmaceutical Companies that Manufacture Thyroid Replacement Hormone and Patient Assistance Programs

Abbott Laboratories/Knoll Pharmaceutical Company
Manufactures: Synthroid
3000 Continental Drive
North Mount Olive, NJ 07828
Telephone (toll-free): 888-566-5506
Patient Assistance Program: Yes. Physician's office should call
1-800-222-6885 (Monday–Friday, 8:00 A.M.–5:00 P.M. CST) to request an application.
Web: www.abbott.com and www.synthroid.com

Forest Laboratories, Inc.
Manufactures: Armour Thyroid, Thyrolar, Levothroid
13600 Shoreline Drive
St. Louis, MO 63045
Telephone (toll-free): 1-800-678-1605
Fax: 314-493-7457
Patient Assistance Program: Yes. Call company for information.
Web: www.frx.com, www.armourthyroid.com, www.levothroid.com, and www.thyrolar.com

King Pharmaceuticals/Jones Pharma
Manufactures: Levoxyl and Cytomel through its wholly-owned subsidiary, Jones Pharma
1945 Craig Road
St. Louis, MO 63146
Telephone (toll-free): 1-800-525-8466
Patient Assistance Program: Yes. Call the company for details.
Web: www.jmedpharma.com and www.kingpharm.com

Mova Pharmaceuticals
Manufactures: Levo-T
Villa Blanca Industrial Park
State Road #1, Km. 34.8
Caguas, Puerto Rico 00725
Telephone (toll-free): 1-800-468-5201
Patient Assistance Program: Call number above.
Web: www.movapharm.com

TogetherRX
A drug card program sponsored by seven drug manufacturers and administered by McKesson, a pharmaceutical distributor. The no-cost card provides discounts to low-income seniors and disabled people.
McKesson Telephone (toll-free):
1-888-4-MBS-BIO
TogetherRX Telephone (toll-free):
1-800-865-7211
Web: www.TogetherRX.com

Watson Pharma, Inc.
Manufactures: Unithroid
Corporate Headquarters
311 Bonnie Circle
Corona, CA 92880
Telephone (toll-free): 1-800-272-5525
Patient Assistance Program: Not for Unithroid.
Web: www.watsonpharm.com and www.unithroid.com

Western Research Laboratories
Manufactures: Westhroid/Naturethroid
21602 North 21st Avenue
Phoenix, AZ 85027
Telephone (toll-free): 1-877-797-7997
Fax: 1-623-879-8683
Patient Assistance Program: No, but assistance through the TogetherRX card program (see above).
Web:
www.westernreasearchlaboratories.com

Web Sites of Further Interest

www.amwa.org
The American Medical Women's Association site contains information related specifically to women and thyroid disease, especially hypothyroidism.

www.aad.org
The American Academy of Dermatology provides information about skin and hair issues arising from thyroid disorders, sponsors Hair Loss Awareness Month each August, and provides a toll-free hotline to give people more information about hair loss treatment options. The number is 1-888-462-DERM.

www.cobrahealth.com
For information about C.O.B.R.A. (Consolidated Omnibus Budget Reconciliation Act).

www.disability.gov
U.S. government site that includes information on living and working with disabilities.

www.elaws.dol.gov/fmla
U.S. government site for the Family and Medical Leave Act.

www.endocrineweb.com
Information on endocrine disorders and endocrine surgery. Provides a doctor search function.

www.fda.gov/cder/drugprepare/KI_Q&A.htm
U.S. Food and Drug Administration site for information about potassium iodide policies and availability.

www.ftc.gov
Site for the Federal Trade Commission and link to the FTC's Operation Cure-All, which gives the facts about effectiveness and problems of health supplements and other products.

www.healthfinder.gov
U.S. government site that provides information about health-related items.

www.icanonline.net
News, information, message boards, and links to Web sites about professional, legal, financial, and emotional aspects of living with disabilities.

www.kidshealth.org
The Nemours Foundation's Web site for parents and prenatal through teenage children. Explains diseases, disorders, and health concerns in user-friendly language.

www.lightoflifefoundation
Dedicated to thyroid cancer patients. Information about causes and treatment, and message boards.

www.Mayoclinic.com
Information on disorders and diseases. Links to related organizations and Web sites.

www.medjetassistance.org
Web site hub of a company that provides medical evacuation and repatriation services if you travel in the United States or abroad.

www.nhlbisupport.com/bmi
Online calculator that computes body mass index (BMI) automatically when you enter your height and weight.

www.nrc.gov/what-we-do/regulatory/emer-resp/emer-prep/ki-faq.html
U.S. Nuclear Regulatory Commission's site for information regarding polices toward and availability of potassium iodide.

www.pubmed.com
Medical database for the latest credible research on disease, conditions, and issues in medicine.

www.snopes.com
Monitors Internet rumors and urban legends and publishes information about their veracity. Good place to go if you hear about a "thyroid cure" or rumors of a better treatment.

www.the-thyroid-society.org
This organization is now part of the American Thyroid Association. Its Web site still has good information on all thyroid-related disorders and treatments.

www.thyroid-fed.org
The Thyroid Federation International's slogan is, "Thyroid Disease in a Global Perspective." This is a cyber gathering place of thyroidologists and patients.

www.thyroidmanager.org
A forum for thyroidologists to communicate their latest findings and comment about the causes and treatments of thyroid disorders. Although this site is geared toward physicians, the thyroid patient can find much useful and interesting information here.

www.usdoj.gov/crt/ada/adahom1.htm
The United States Department of Justice Americans with Disabilities Act Home Page. Includes information about the ADA, news, and links to other federal government agencies with ADA responsibilities.

www.webmed.com
A general health site with links to specific disease, disorder, and information sites and pamphlets.

Acknowledgments

THERE ARE many people who have contributed to the writing of this book, and I am very grateful to them. My first thanks go to the doctors and other medical professionals "on the front lines," who took time out of their busy days to answer my questions, provide guidance, and review my work. These amazing individuals include: David Hallegua, M.D.; Elliot G. Levy, M.D., Basil Rapoport, M.B.; Lisa Waldman; Daniel J. Wallace, M.D., and Donald Wood, M.D.

My great appreciation goes to Edie Stern of the American Thyroid Association for her support and review of some of the material in this book, and to Kevin R. Laverty of The Thyroid Foundation of America, Inc., for his guidance and help. Also, my thanks to Tess Baldwin, R.Ph., and Kirk, whose help navigating pharmaceutical information was invaluable!

I am very thankful for the insight of the hypothyroid patients and their loved ones with whom I spoke and whose "words of wisdom" are included in this book. Diana, Mir, Lyn, David, Carol, Jo Ann, Ed, and Joyce—you are inspirations! And I'm also beholden to Donal Koehane for his illustration and Frank Desiderio, C.S.P., for his perspective on healing and prayer.

ACKNOWLEDGMENTS

The people who brought this book into being are remarkable. Jane Jordan Browne, Matthew Lore, Sue McCloskey, Howard Grossman, Pauline Neuwirth, and the whole team at Marlowe & Company—thank you for opening this opportunity up to me and seeing it from start to finish. It's been a wonderful journey!

Index